Urologic Cancer: Endoscopic, Laparoscopic, and Robot-Assisted Surgery Management

Urologic Cancer: Endoscopic, Laparoscopic, and Robot-Assisted Surgery Management

Guest Editor

Kouji Izumi

MDPI

Basel • Beijing • Wuhan • Barcelona • Belgrade • Novi Sad • Cluj • Manchester

Guest Editor
Kouji Izumi
Department of Integrative
Cancer Therapy and Urology
Kanazawa University
Graduate School of
Medical Science
Ishikawa
Japan

Editorial Office
MDPI AG
Grosspeteranlage 5
4052 Basel, Switzerland

This is a reprint of the Special Issue, published open access by the journal *Cancers* (ISSN 2072-6694), freely accessible at: https://www.mdpi.com/journal/cancers/special_issues/Robot_Assisted_Surgery.

For citation purposes, cite each article independently as indicated on the article page online and as indicated below:

Lastname, A.A.; Lastname, B.B. Article Title. *Journal Name* **Year**, *Volume Number*, Page Range.

ISBN 978-3-7258-6866-7 (Hbk)
ISBN 978-3-7258-6867-4 (PDF)
https://doi.org/10.3390/books978-3-7258-6867-4

Contents

About the Editor

Kouji Izumi

Kouji Izumi is not only a board-certified urologist of the Japanese Urological Association but also a medical oncologist, serving as a board-certified senior member of the Japanese Society of Medical Oncology. As a basic researcher, he has published numerous studies on immune tolerance within the cancer microenvironment, with particular focus on tumor-associated macrophages and cytokines in prostate, kidney, and bladder cancers. He spent two years as a research associate at the George Whipple Laboratory for Cancer Research at the University of Rochester, Rochester, NY, where he investigated the relationship between the androgen receptor and the immune system. He earned his PhD from Kanazawa University for his work on the acquisition of castration resistance in prostate cancer.

As a urologist, he is certified in urinary laparoscopic technology by the Japanese Society of Endourology and Robotics and holds endoscopic surgical skill qualification from the Japan Society of Endoscopic Surgery. He has been engaged in robotic surgery for 15 years and holds proctor and mentor certifications for both the da Vinci and Hinotori robot-assisted surgical systems. Dr. Izumi has received multiple academic awards, including the Research Award of the 19th Japanese Association for Metastasis Research (2015), the Academic Award of the Japanese Society of Endourology and Robotics (2022), and the Best Poster Award at the European Society for Medical Oncology Asia 2025.

Preface

Recent advances in robot-assisted urologic surgery have significantly improved the quality of life for patients with prostate, bladder, and kidney cancers by enabling less-invasive procedures, reducing blood loss, and preserving functional outcomes. These developments may also influence diagnostic value; however, their overall impact remains insufficiently evaluated due to limited data and short follow-up periods. This Special Issue, including 10 papers, features state-of-the-art studies not only on robot-assisted urologic surgery but also on laparoscopic and transurethral approaches.

Nakagawa et al. investigated bladder cancers presenting with the inchworm sign to clarify factors associated with muscle-invasive disease and to assess its prognostic value. Among 109 patients, they found that 86.2% had non-muscle invasive bladder cancer, while non-papillary morphology and bladder-neck location strongly predicted muscle invasion. They also compared outcomes in non-muscle invasive bladder cancer with and without the inchworm sign and observed no significant differences in recurrence-free or progression-free survival. Positive urine cytology was the only prognostic factor for recurrence. These findings help clinicians better interpret the inchworm sign and identify patients at risk for muscle-invasive disease.

Kawaguchi et al. investigated outcomes of robot-assisted partial nephrectomy (RAPN) and percutaneous cryoablation for small-renal-cell carcinomas in elderly patients. Analyzing 99 individuals aged 70 years or older, they found that major perioperative complications were rare, occurring in only one RAPN case. Both treatments resulted in postoperative declines in renal function, while recurrence-free and overall survival tended to be better with RAPN, though not significantly. The study suggests that RAPN is a safe and effective option for elderly patients, and that percutaneous cryoablation serves as a valuable alternative for those at high risk for general anesthesia.

Brassetti et al. investigated outcomes of sutureless versus renorrhaphy off-clamp robotic partial nephrectomy for cT1–2 renal masses using a retrospective cohort and propensity score matching. Among 531 patients, the sutureless technique achieved a significantly higher trifecta rate than renorrhaphy, while chronic kidney disease stage migration–free survival was comparable between groups. Age, high RENAL score, and use of renorrhaphy independently predicted lower trifecta achievement. Age and baseline estimated glomerular filtration rate predicted chronic kidney disease progression. These findings suggest that the sutureless approach may improve surgical quality without compromising renal functional outcomes, supporting its use in selected patients.

Zeuschner et al. investigated the cost implications of open retroperitoneal versus robot-assisted transperitoneal partial nephrectomy, focusing particularly on nursing workload as a potential source of savings. Analyzing 259 cases over two years, they found that robotic surgery significantly reduced total and daily nursing time, resulting in meaningful savings in nursing costs and reduced use of erythrocyte concentrates. However, these savings were insufficient to offset the substantially higher material costs of the robotic system, leading to greater overall expenses per case. This study helps clarify the economic trade-offs of robotic partial nephrectomy and informs cost-conscious surgical decision-making.

Gloger et al. investigated risk factors for lymphocele formation after robot-assisted radical prostatectomy and pelvic lymphadenectomy using data from the multicenter ProLy randomized trial. Their multivariate analysis showed that higher BMI, longer surgical time, and study group assignment were independent predictors of lymphocele development. Symptomatic lymphoceles were particularly associated with BMI $\geq$ 30 kg/m^2 and greater intraoperative blood loss. These findings highlight obesity and operative duration as key contributors to postoperative lymphocele risk, helping clinicians identify high-risk patients and optimize perioperative management.

Bislev et al. investigated oncological outcomes in patients with low-grade upper tract urothelial carcinoma treated with endoscopic laser ablation. Analyzing 118 consecutive cases over a 10-year period, they found a high rate of local recurrence, with most recurrences occurring within the first three years. Despite this, progression was rare, and overall and disease-specific survival remained high at both two and five years. These findings indicate that laser ablation is a safe treatment option for low-grade upper tract urothelial carcinoma, while emphasizing the need for close and frequent follow-up to detect early recurrence.

Feciche et al. The authors reviewed the current evidence on posterior retroperitoneal laparoscopic adrenalectomy (PRLA), examining its anatomical basis, surgical technique, and clinical implications. They describe the "backdoor" retroperitoneal approach and outline key technical steps, including patient positioning, trocar placement, and adrenal dissection. Their analysis shows that PRLA offers reduced postoperative pain, shorter hospitalization, and faster recovery compared with open surgery, while maintaining comparable oncological outcomes in appropriately selected patients. Although the technique requires familiarity with posterior anatomy and presents spatial challenges, the findings support PRLA as a safe and effective alternative to traditional adrenalectomy, helping guide surgical decision-making and future refinement.

Zohar et al. investigated a refined surgical technique for robotic radical nephroureterectomy using the da Vinci Xi platform, focusing on a one-docking, three-port approach. Analyzing 15 consecutive cases performed by a single surgeon, they found that the technique enabled efficient multi-quadrant dissection with a median operative time of 133 minutes and low blood loss. Complication rates were acceptable, and lymph node dissection did not prolong surgery. Their findings demonstrate that combining minimal port usage with the Xi system's camera-hop feature provides a safe and effective method for robotic radical nephroureterectomy, helping streamline complex procedures and improve operative efficiency.

Reitano et al. systematically reviewed the feasibility, safety, and reproducibility of Da Vinci Single-Port robot-assisted adrenalectomy (DV-SP RAA). Across five retrospective studies including 342 patients, DV-SP RAA demonstrated short operative times, low estimated blood loss, and very low complication rates. Most procedures were completed through a single incision, and cosmetic outcomes were superior to those of multi-port approaches. Comparative analyses showed no increase in perioperative risk. Although limited by small sample sizes and selection bias, the findings suggest that DV-SP RAA is a promising minimally invasive technique that may guide future clinical adoption and research.

Chang et al. investigated whether robotic radical nephroureterectomy (RARNU) offers oncologic or perioperative advantages over laparoscopic radical nephroureterectomy (LRNU) for upper tract urothelial carcinoma (UTUC). In this large multicenter retrospective study of 2037 patients, overlap weighting and multiple imputations were used to balance baseline characteristics. After adjustment, RARNU and LRNU demonstrated comparable rates of complications, residual tumor, disease recurrence, and UTUC-related mortality, with similar overall, cancer-specific, and disease-free survival. These findings indicate that RARNU provides outcomes equivalent to LRNU and may help surgeons—especially those with limited laparoscopic experience—adopt minimally invasive RNU more easily.

Together, these studies highlight the rapid evolution of minimally invasive urologic surgery and provide valuable insights that will help refine clinical decision-making and improve patient outcomes worldwide. I hope that this collection inspires urologists across the globe to continue advancing the field with innovation, precision, and compassion.

Kouji Izumi
Guest Editor

cancers MDPI

Article

Does Bladder Cancer with Inchworm Sign Indicate Better Prognosis after TURBT?

Ryunosuke Nakagawa [1], Kouji Izumi [1,*], Renato Naito [1], Suguru Kadomoto [1], Hiroaki Iwamoto [1], Hiroshi Yaegashi [1], Shohei Kawaguchi [1], Takahiro Nohara [1], Kazuyoshi Shigehara [1], Kotaro Yoshida [2], Yoshifumi Kadono [1] and Atsushi Mizokami [1]

[1] Department of Integrative Cancer Therapy and Urology, Kanazawa University Graduate School of Medical Science, Kanazawa 920-8641, Japan

[2] Department of Radiology, Kanazawa University Graduate School of Medical Science, Kanazawa 920-8641, Japan

* Correspondence: kouji1974@staff.kanazawa-u.ac.jp; Tel.: +81-76-265-2393; Fax: +81-76-234-4263

Simple Summary: Inchworm sign is considered to be a characteristic finding in non-muscle invasive bladder cancer. We retrospectively investigated the factors related to muscle invasive status in bladder cancer associated with inchworm sign and the role of inchworm sign in tumor outcomes following transurethral resection of bladder tumor. Of the 109 patients with inchworm sign, 94 (86.2%) were non-muscle invasive bladder cancer. Non-papillary tumors and tumors located in the bladder neck were significant predictors of muscle invasive bladder cancer with inchworm sign. Additionally, inchworm sign was not a prognostic factor in patients with non-muscle invasive bladder cancer in this study.

Abstract: Background: Inchworm sign is considered to be a characteristic finding in non-muscle invasive bladder cancer (NMIBC). Nevertheless, pathologically diagnosed muscle invasive bladder cancers (MIBCs) are occasionally diagnosed from tissue obtained by transurethral resection of bladder tumor (TURBT) in patients with inchworm sign. Methods: We retrospectively investigated the factors related to muscle invasive status in bladder cancer associated with inchworm sign and the role of inchworm sign in tumor outcomes following TURBT. Results: Of the 109 patients with inchworm sign, 94 (86.2%) and 15 (13.8%) were NMIBC and MIBC, respectively. Non-papillary tumors (hazard ratio (HR): 9.55, 95% confidence interval (CI): 2.07–44.10; $p < 0.01$) and tumors located in the bladder neck (HR: 7.73, 95% CI: 1.83–32.76; $p < 0.01$) were significant predictors of MIBC in bladder cancer with inchworm sign. Furthermore, recurrence-free survival (RFS) and progression-free survival were compared between patients with NMIBC with and without inchworm sign; however, no significant differences were found. In patients with NMIBC with inchworm sign, positive urine cytology was a prognostic factor for RFS (HR: 1.90, 95% CI: 1.04–3.48; $p = 0.04$). Conclusions: In bladder cancer with inchworm sign, 86.2% were NMIBC. Even in the case of inchworm sign, the presence of a non-papillary tumor or a bladder neck tumor before TURBT should be noted because of the possibility of MIBC. In this study, the inchworm sign was not a prognostic factor in patients with NMIBC.

Keywords: inchworm sign; non-invasive muscle bladder cancer; muscle invasive bladder cancer; bladder neck; non-papillary tumor

1. Introduction

Bladder cancer (BC) is the tenth most commonly diagnosed cancer, and the age-standardized incidence rate (per 100,000 person-years) is 9.5 for men and 2.4 for women worldwide [1]. Treatment for BC depends on the stage of the disease; however, the degree of cancer invasion is one of the most important factors [2]. While total cystectomy is the standard treatment for BC that has invaded the muscle layer, which is called muscle invasive bladder cancer (MIBC), non-muscle invasive bladder cancer (NMIBC) is likely to be treated by follow-up or bladder-preservation options, such as Bacille Calmette–Guerin (BCG), depending on the risk [3]. Transurethral resection of bladder tumor (TURBT) is commonly performed for BC not only for therapeutic but also for diagnostic purposes, and the pathological results are used to determine treatment options [2–4]. Moreover, it is useful for predicting cancer invasion by preoperative imaging evaluation. Panebianco et al. established an imaging protocol using multi-parametric magnetic resonance imaging (MRI), called VI-RADS, to classify and evaluate the risk of muscle invasion into five categories [5]. Underdiagnosis by TURBT is often a challenge [6]; however, standardization of imaging evaluation and prediction of muscle layer invasion may prevent it.

Diffusion-weighted imaging (DWI) is constructed by quantifying the diffusion of the water molecules in tissues and is excellent in the delineation of BC [7], and the signal reflects the characteristics of the tumor tissue [8]. DWI is more accurate than T2-weighted MRI in BC staging, particularly in staging-localized lesions of pT1–2 [9]. The "inchworm sign" in DWI, proposed by Takeuchi et al., is reported to predict NMIBC [10]. They suggested that inchworm sign showed a bow-shaped tumor with high signal intensity and a submucosal stalk with low signal intensity on DWI. They also reported that the inchworm sign was a characteristic finding in all 28 pT1 cases studied and was useful in differentiating MIBC.

In this study, we focused on the inchworm sign and investigated the factors related to muscle invasive status in BC with inchworm sign and the role of the inchworm sign in tumor outcomes following TURBT.

2. Patients and Methods

2.1. Patient Selection and Collection of Clinical Data

Among the patients with BC receiving treatment at Kanazawa University Hospital from 2007 to 2019, those with BC without metastasis and with inchworm sign on DWI were included in this study. Only initial cases were included, and recurrent cases were not included. Cases with multiple tumors were included. Patients who did not have an MRI at diagnosis or had an MRI but no DWI were excluded. We also excluded cases with coexisting upper tract urothelial carcinoma at the initial diagnosis. The probability of NMIBC and predictors of MIBC in these patients with BC were retrospectively investigated. The inchworm sign is defined as a finding on diffusion-weighted (DW)-MRI that shows a bow-shaped tumor with high signal intensity and a submucosal stalk with low signal intensity.

Moreover, patients with NMIBC who had an MRI at diagnosis were selected and categorized into two groups with and without inchworm sign. The recurrence-free survival (RFS) and progression-free survival (PFS) of both groups were compared. RFS was measured from the diagnosis of BC to recurrence or last follow-up. PFS was measured from the diagnosis of BC until recurrence of MIBC or appearance of metastasis or last follow-up. Follow-up was terminated on March 2022. Clinical stage was determined based on the eighth edition of the Union for International Cancer Control Tumor, Node, and Metastasis classification published on 2017.

2.2. Image Analysis

A single urologist with 7 years of experience in reading abdominal DWI data and performing TURBT (Reviewer 1) reviewed the MR images blinded to the clinical and histologic information. The tumor image with high signal intensity and a submucosal stalk with low signal intensity on DWI were identified as positive for the inchworm sign. To ensure interobserver concordance in assessment of the inchworm sign, one reviewer (Reviewer 2—a radiologist with 19 years of experience reading abdominal DWI data), who did not disclose the clinical course and histological findings, independently evaluated the presence of inchworm signs on all images.

2.3. Statistical Analyses

Binomial logistic regression analysis was used to evaluate the predictive impact of potential factors of MIBC in patients with positive inchworm sign. The Cox proportional hazards model was used to evaluate the predictive impact of potential factors of RFS and PFS. All factors were divided into dichotomized variable categories and evaluated. Hazard ratios (HRs) and 95% confidence intervals (CIs) were calculated. RFS and PFS were estimated using the Kaplan–Meier method, with differences being compared using log-rank tests. Statistical analyses were performed using the commercially available software Prism 8 (GraphPad, San Diego, CA, USA) and SPSS ver. 25.0 (SPSS Inc, Chicago, IL, USA), with p values of <0.05 indicating statistical significance.

2.4. Ethical Considerations

This study was approved by the Institutional Review Board of Kanazawa University Hospital (2021-300). Informed consent was obtained in the form of opt-out posted at our facility allowed by the Medical Ethics Committee of Kanazawa University. All methods were performed in accordance with the relevant guidelines and regulations.

3. Results

3.1. Patient Characteristics with Inchworm Sign

A representative inchworm sign, showing a bow-shaped tumor with high signal intensity and a submucosal stalk with low signal intensity on DW-MRI, is shown in Figure 1.

The characteristics of the patients with BC with inchworm sign on DW-MRI are presented in Table 1. A total of 109 patients were identified with inchworm sign. Regarding pT stage, 2 (1.8%), 48 (44.0%), 44 (40.4%), and 14 (13.8%) patients were Tis, Ta, T1, and T2 and above, respectively. A total of 94 (86.2%) patients had NMIBC. Additionally, 38 (34.9%), 92 (84.4%), 46 (42.2%), 82 (75.2%), and 73 (67.0%) patients had a tumor size of >30 mm, papillary tumors, multiple tumors, hematuria, and positive urine cytology, respectively. The most frequent tumor location was the lateral wall (54.1%). There was a total of 37 surgeons in the 12-year period, due to staff transitions at our facility. All surgeons were similar in terms of surgical techniques. For surgical instruments, an Olympus TURis bipolar resectoscope (Olympus Corporation, Tokyo, Japan) was used, and an Aladuck LS-DLED (SBI Pharma, Tokyo, Japan) or Storz PDD system and Storz bipolar resectoscope (KARL STORZ, Tuttlingen, Germany) was used for photodynamic diagnosis (PDD)-TURBT. Twenty-one patients (19.3%) received immediate postoperative intravesical chemotherapy. The drugs administered varied from pirarubicin, mitomycin C, and epirubicin hydrochloride.

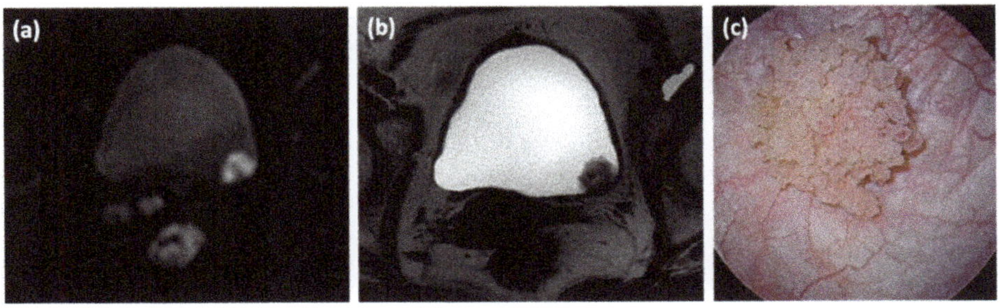

Figure 1. The case of bladder cancer with inchworm sign. Findings of bladder cancer in a 72-year-old woman diagnosed with hematuria. (**a**) Diffusion-weighted (DW)-MRI shows high signal intensity from the tumor and low signal intensity from the submucosal stalk. This finding is defined as the inchworm sign. (**b**) Transverse T2-weighted MRI shows a tumor on the left lateral wall of the bladder; however, no change in the internal signal intensity is observed. (**c**) Cystoscopy reveals a papillary tumor at the same site.

Table 1. Characteristics of the patients with inchworm sign.

Variable		
No. of patients		109
Age (median)		71
Sex		
	Male (%)	90 (82.6)
	Female (%)	19 (17.4)
Histology		
	UC (%)	94 (86.2)
	UC with squamous differentiation (%)	10 (9.2)
	UC with glandular differentiation (%)	5 (4.6)
Pathological grade		
	1 (%)	4 (3.7)
	2 (%)	65 (59.6)
	3 (%)	30 (27.5)
	Unknown (%)	10 (9.2)
pT stage		
	Tis (%)	2 (1.8)
	Ta (%)	48 (44.0)
	T1 (%)	44 (40.4)
	T2 (%)	11 (10.1)
	T3 (%)	2 (1.8)
	T4 (%)	2 (1.8)
Tumor size		
	10–30 mm (%)	71 (65.1)
	30 mm < (%)	38 (34.9)
Tumor location		
	Anterior wall (%)	13 (11.9)
	Posterior wall (%)	17 (15.6)
	Side wall (%)	59 (54.1)
	Dome (%)	3 (2.8)
	Neck (%)	17 (15.6)
Papillary		
	Yes (%)	92 (84.4)
	No (%)	17 (15.6)
Multiple tumors		
	Yes (%)	46 (42.2)
	No (%)	63 (57.8)
Hematuria		
	Yes (%)	82 (75.2)
	No (%)	26 (23.9)
	Unknown (%)	1 (0.9)
Cytology		
	Negative (%)	36 (33.0)
	Positive (%)	73 (67.0)

3.2. Predictors of MIBC in Patients with Inchworm Sign

We examined the predictors of MIBC in patients with inchworm sign. In univariate analysis, multiple tumors (HR: 3.22, 95% CI: 1.02–10.19; $p = 0.04$), tumor size >30 mm (HR: 6.82, 95% CI: 1.99–23.31; $p < 0.01$), non-papillary tumors (HR: 5.03, 95% CI: 1.50–16.86; $p < 0.01$), and location in the bladder neck (HR: 10.79, 95% CI: 3.17–36.75; $p < 0.01$) were predictive factors for MIBC (Table 2). In multivariable analysis, non-papillary tumors (HR: 9.55, 95% CI: 2.07–44.10; $p < 0.01$) and localization to the bladder neck (HR: 7.73, 95% CI: 1.83–32.76; $p < 0.01$) were significant predictive factors for MIBC. The cases with non-papillary tumor (Figure 2a–c) and bladder neck tumor (Figure 2d–f) with inchworm sign but which are MIBC are shown in Figure 2.

Table 2. Predictors of MIBC in patients with positive inchworm sign.

Variables	Univariate				Multivariable			
	95% CI *p* Value	HR	Lower	Upper	95% CI *p* Value	HR	Lower	Upper
Age ≥ 75 (years)	0.49	1.48	0.49	4.42				
Female	0.72	0.75	0.15	3.65				
Cytology positive	0.15	3.12	0.65	14.89				
Hematuria	0.65	1.37	0.36	5.28				
Multiple tumors	0.04	3.22	1.02	10.19	0.09	3.38	0.83	13.69
Tumor size >30 mm	<0.01	6.82	1.99	23.31	0.053	4.27	0.98	18.64
Non-papillary tumor	<0.01	5.03	1.50	16.86	<0.01	9.55	2.07	44.10
Bladder neck	<0.01	10.79	3.17	36.75	<0.01	7.73	1.83	32.76

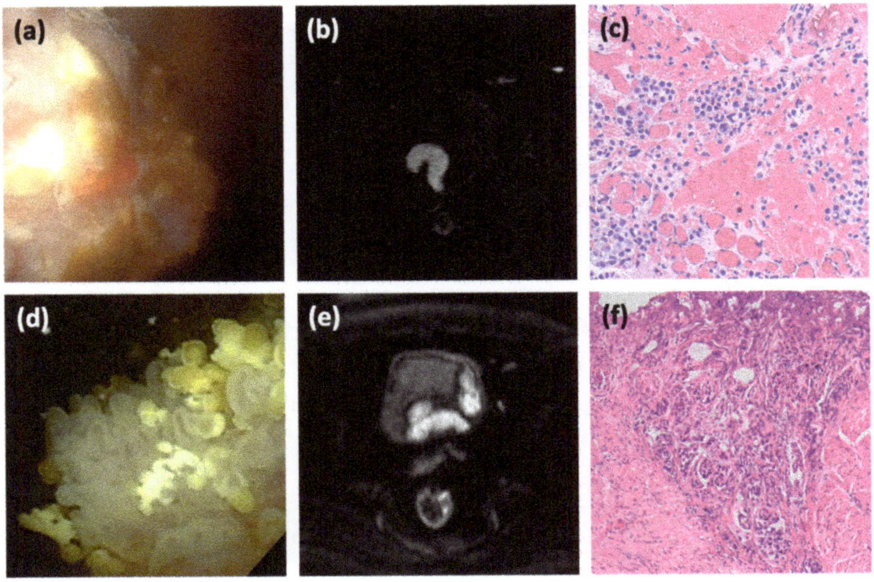

Figure 2. Bladder cancer with muscle invasion despite the presence of inchworm sign. A 77-year-old man consulted for hematuria (**a–c**). Cystoscopy shows a non-papillary tumor on the right wall (**a**); DW-MRI shows the inchworm sign (**b**); and TURBT shows tumor invasion into the muscle layer, and the diagnosis of MIBC was made (**c**). A 76-year-old man referred for urinary frequency and gross hematuria (**d–f**). Cystoscopy reveals a papillary tumor in the neck (**d**). MRI shows a bladder tumor with inchworm sign and multiple tumors on the lateral wall of the bladder (**e**). The resected tissue of the neck tumor shows findings of muscle invasion (**f**).

3.3. RFS and PFS Stratified by the Presence of Inchworm Sign on Patients with NMIBC

Subsequently, patients with NMIBC (Ta and T1) with and without inchworm sign were grouped. A total of 77 patients with NMIBC without inchworm sign and 92 with inchworm sign were noted. The characteristics of patients with NMIBC are shown in Table 3. NMIBC with inchworm sign had significantly higher percentages of a tumor size >30 mm ($p < 0.01$), positive cytology ($p = 0.03$), and pT1 ($p = 0.01$). Comparison of RFS (HR: 1.49, 95% CI: 0.98–2.27; $p = 0.06$) and PFS (HR: 1.92, 95% CI: 0.62–5.96; $p = 0.28$) between the two groups showed no significant difference (Figure 3). Furthermore, we compared RFS and PFS for each patient with pTa and pT1, respectively, and found no significant differences (Figure 4).

Table 3. Characteristics of patients with NMIBC.

Variable		Inchworm Sign −	Inchworm Sign +	*p* Value
No. of patients		77	92	
Age (median)		73	71	0.35
Sex				0.75
	Male (%)	65 (84.4)	76 (82.6)	
	Female (%)	12 (15.6)	16 (17.4)	
Tumor size				<0.01
	10–30 mm (%)	72 (98.7)	65 (64.9)	
	>30 mm (%)	5 (1.3)	27 (35.1)	
Multiple tumors				0.42
	Yes (%)	34 (44.2)	35 (38.0)	
	No (%)	43 (55.8)	57 (62.0)	
Histology				0.66
	UC (%)	71 (92.2)	81 (88.0)	
	UC with squamous differentiation (%)	2 (2.6)	4 (4.3)	
	UC with glandular differentiation (%)	4 (5.2)	7 (8.7)	
Pathological grade				0.11
	1 (%)	9 (11.7)	4 (4.3)	
	2 (%)	45 (58.4)	61 (66.3)	
	3 (%)	11 (14.3)	19 (20.7)	
	Unknown (%)	12 (15.6)	8 (8.7)	
Cytology				0.03
	Negative (%)	38 (49.4)	34 (37.0)	
	Positive (%)	33 (42.9)	56 (60.9)	
	Unknown (%)	6 (16.5)	2 (2.1)	
pT stage				0.01
	Ta (%)	53 (68.8)	44 (47.8)	
	T1 (%)	24 (31.2)	48 (52.2)	
BCG treatment				0.39
	Yes (%)	15 (19.5)	23 (25.0)	
	No (%)	62 (80.5)	69 (75.0)	
PDD				0.13
	Yes (%)	3 (3.9)	9 (9.8)	
	No (%)	74 (96.1)	82 (90.2)	

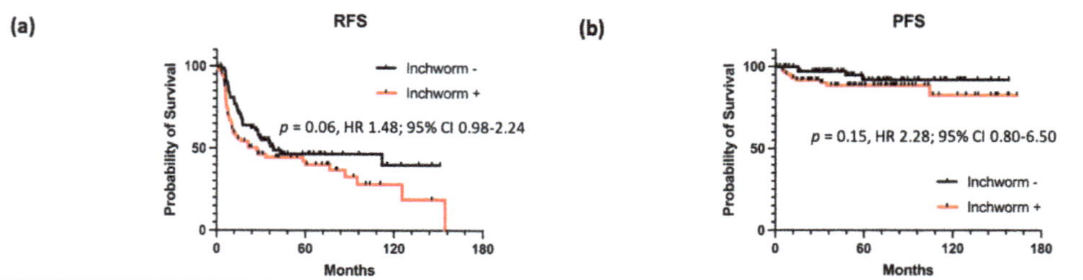

	Median RFS	Numbers at risk		
Inchworm -	38.4	77	16	4
Inchworm +	26.6	92	18	3

	Median PFS	Numbers at risk		
Inchworm -	NR	77	33	10
Inchworm +	NR	92	41	12

Figure 3. Kaplan-Meier survival curves for recurrence-free survival. (**a**) Progression−free survival. (**b**) Stratified by the presence of inchworm sign for patients with NMIBC. Comparison of RFS (HR: 1.49, 95% CI: 0.98–2.27; $p = 0.06$) and PFS (HR: 1.92, 95% CI: 0.62–5.96; $p = 0.28$) between the negative and positive inchworm sign groups shows no significant difference.

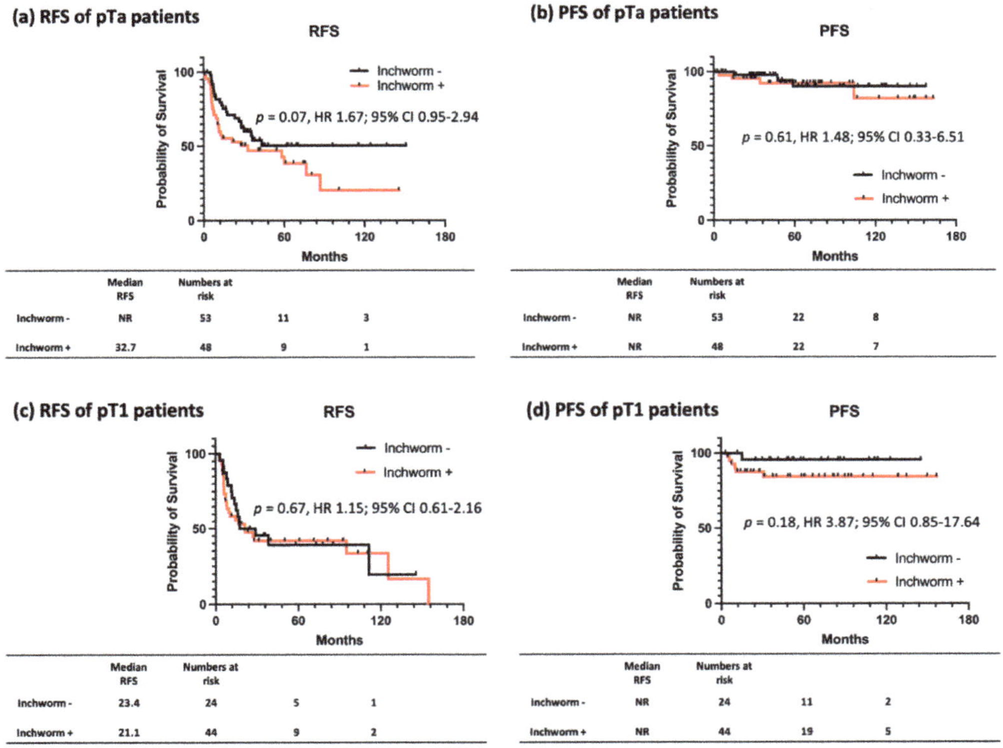

Figure 4. Kaplan-Meier survival curves for recurrence-free survival and progression-free survival stratified by the presence of an inchworm sign for patients with pTa and pT1. Patients with NMIBC are compared for RFS and PFS with and without inchworm sign in pTa and pT1. In patients with pTa, RFS tends to be worse in those with inchworm sign; however, the difference is not significant (**a**). No other comparisons are significantly different (**b–d**).

3.4. Prognostic Factors for RFS and PFS of Patients with NMIBC with/without Inchworm Sign

We focused on patients with NMIBC with inchworm sign and investigated the prognostic factors for RFS and PFS. We identified positive cytology (HR: 1.90, 95% CI: 1.04–3.48; $p = 0.04$) as a predictor for RFS (Table 4). Conversely, no prognostic factors for PFS were found (Table 4). Furthermore, prognostic factors for RFS and PFS in patients with NMIBC without inchworm sign were investigated. However, positive cytology (HR: 1.60, 95% CI: 0.80–3.22; $p = 0.19$) was not a predictor for RFS, and only multiple tumors (HR: 3.04, 95% CI: 1.56–5.90; $p > 0.01$) was the prognostic factor (Table 5). No prognostic factors for PFS were noted (Table 5).

3.5. Interobserver Variability in Identification of Inchworm Sign

We assessed interobserver variability in the identification of inchworm signs. Reviewers 1 and 2 independently analyzed the DW images of all eligible tumors and found inchworm signs in 108 (33.2%) and 112 (34.5%) tumors, respectively. Interobserver variability between the two readers was generally excellent, with a kappa coefficient of 0.85.

Table 4. Univariate analysis of the prognostic factors for recurrence-free survival and progression-free survival of patients with NMIBC with positive inchworm sign.

(a) RFS					(b) PFS				
Variables	*p* Value	HR	95% CI Lower	Upper	Variables	*p* Value	HR	95% CI Lower	Upper
Age ≥ 75 (years)	0.39	0.78	0.44	1.38	Age ≥ 75 (years)	0.72	1.27	0.36	4.53
Male	0.67	1.18	0.55	2.52	Male	0.43	2.29	0.29	18.09
Tumor size ≥ 30 mm	0.81	1.08	0.6	1.93	Tumor size ≥ 30 mm	0.15	2.51	0.73	8.72
Bladder neck	0.92	0.95	0.38	2.4	Bladder neck	0.5	0.04	>0.01	440.34
Non-papillary tumor	0.41	0.61	0.19	1.97	Non-papillary tumor	0.52	0.04	>0.01	573.38
Multiple tumors	0.29	0.74	0.42	1.3	Multiple tumors	0.58	0.68	0.18	2.64
Hematuria	0.66	1.15	0.61	2.17	Hematuria	0.25	3.38	0.43	26.8
Positive cytology	0.04	1.9	1.04	3.48	Positive cytology	0.15	47.15	0.25	9005.87
BCG treatment	0.82	0.93	0.48	1.8	BCG treatment	0.16	2.48	0.7	8.8
PDD	0.27	0.45	0.11	1.86	PDD	0.58	0.04	>0.01	2761.93

Table 5. Univariate analysis of the prognostic factors for recurrence-free survival and progression-free survival of patients with NMIBC with negative inchworm sign.

(a) RFS					(b) PFS				
Variables	*p* Value	HR	95% CI Lower	Upper	Variables	*p* Value	HR	95% CI Lower	Upper
Age ≥ 75 (years)	0.13	1.64	0.86	3.14	Age ≥ 75 (years)	0.65	0.6	0.06	5.71
Male	0.28	1.78	0.63	5.07	Male	0.7	0.64	0.07	6.27
Tumor size ≥ 30 mm	0.09	2.83	0.85	9.34					
Bladder neck	0.47	0.65	0.2	2.12					
Non-papillary tumor	0.33	1.51	0.66	3.48	Non-papillary tumor	0.55	0.04	>0.01	1955.36
Multiple tumors	>0.01	3.04	1.56	5.9	Multiple tumors	0.5	0.46	0.05	4.39
Hematuria	0.7	1.14	0.59	2.17	Hematuria	0.99	0.98	0.14	7
Positive cytology	0.19	1.6	0.8	3.22	Positive cytology	0.21	4.28	0.44	41.43
BCG treatment	0.46	1.33	0.63	2.82	BCG treatment	0.82	1.31	0.14	12.63
PDD	0.88	1.12	0.27	4.69					

4. Discussion

In this study, 86.2% of patients with BC with inchworm sign were NMIBC. Saito et al. reported that the stalk extending from the bladder wall to the tumor center is composed of fibrous tissue, capillaries, inflammatory cells, and edema [11]. Takeuchi et al. also reported that pT1 bladder cancer with inchworm sign histologically has a submucosal stalk consisting of significantly edematous submucosa, fibrous tissue, capillaries, and mild inflammatory cell infiltration, which is consistent with a low signal intensity region on DW-MRI, and is one of the indicators in the imaging findings of NMIBC [10]. Although there are no reports on the formation of the inchworm sign, we suspect that the thickening of the submucosa due to inflammation and edema results in the formation of this bow-shaped structure. The probability that BC with inchworm sign indicates NMIBC is high and is considered to be useful in differentiating from MIBC. However, in our study, not all patients with BC with inchworm sign had NMIBC, and 13.8% were diagnosed with MIBC. Kobayashi et al. reported that 25% of patients diagnosed with NMIBC based on the findings of inchworm sign were consequently pathologically diagnosed with MIBC [12]. They suggested that the fading images of surrounding tissues in DW-MRI may result in loss of anatomical information and compromise the staging performance, and they reported that incorporating quantitative information on apparent diffusion coefficient (ADC) values improved the accuracy of inchworm sign staging and greatly reduced the misdiagnosis rate.

We investigated patients with pathologically diagnosed MIBC despite the presence of inchworm sign and found that non-papillary tumor and localization to the bladder neck were predictive factors for MIBC by multivariable analysis. Non-papillary tumors, including nodular tumors, tend to be more malignant and have more muscle layer invasion than papillary tumors [13]. Notably, if the cystoscopy shows a non-papillary tumor, MIBC is highly likely, regardless of the presence or absence of inchworm sign. The trigone muscle presents from the deltoid to the proximal urethra, which may have functional implications for understanding the mechanisms of continence at the bladder neck [14], and the muscular layer gradually thickens from the deltoid to the proximal urethra, while the submucosal tissue becomes occupied and thin [15]. In other words, the bladder neck has a higher percentage of muscle layers. Xiao et al. reported that bladder neck tumors have significantly more muscle layer invasion and an advanced tumor stage at diagnosis, lymphovascular invasion, and higher frequency of local and distant metastases than non-bladder neck tumors [16]. We suggest that MIBC may not be ruled out even if the inchworm sign is observed.

In our study, we found no significant difference in RFS and PFS in patients with NMIBC with or without inchworm sign. Huan-Jun et al. reported that the median diameter of tumors with stems (21.5 mm) was significantly larger than that of tumors without stems (13.0 mm) [17]. They also postulated that submucosal enhancement and stalks are related to the size of the tumors and small tumors may not generate enough pulling force to form stalks. In our study, this may be related to the significantly larger tumor size in NMIBC patients with inchworm sign. Since the percentage of T1 was significantly higher in patients with inchworm sign, Ta and T1 were examined separately; however, no significant difference was observed. Yajima et al. reported that patients with T1 without the inchworm sign had a significantly lower PFS than those with the inchworm sign [18]. Conversely, they also reported no significant difference in RFS. Several reports have suggested that the degree of tumor invasion into the submucosal lamina propria is associated with the progression [19–21], and they proposed that the inchworm sign is one of the indicators that can easily assess the degree of invasion. The reason for the difference between our results and those of Yajima et al. is the lower BCG treatment and the second TURBT (6 of 63 cases, data are not shown) rates in our patients. These factors may impact patient prognosis. Furthermore, we identified a higher rate of positive cytology in patients with NMIBC with inchworm sign, and this factor is strongly associated with worse RFS. Jancke et al. found that a high-grade malignant bladder wash cytology at the primary diagnosis was predictive of recurrence and suggested that this could be considered in designing future follow-up schedules [22]. Furthermore, Kiyoshima et al. reported that patients with BC with a positive cytology had larger tumor diameters and that patients with a positive cytology tended to have shorter RFS [23]. However, in our study, positive cytology was a prognostic factor for worse RFS only in patients with inchworm sign; additionally, tumor size was not a significant factor regardless of the presence or absence of inchworm sign. We hypothesize that this result was due to the surface area of the tumor. A submucosal stalk with low signal intensity on DW-MRI in the inchworm sign indicates a stalked tumor; the surface area of a tumor with an inchworm sign may be larger than that of a tumor without an inchworm sign with the same length (Figure 5). This difference in surface area may have affected the higher positive urinary cytology rate in patients with inchworm sign and, consequently, may have been a prognostic factor for RFS. In addition, cancer cells in BC with the inchworm sign may have a higher tendency to segregate from the tumor. These structural differences may also explain why patients with pTa with inchworm sign tended to have worse RFS. The surface area of tumors with inchworm sign is an issue that requires further investigation.

This study has several limitations. First, this study was retrospective, and the evaluation of treatment effects was left to individual physicians, which may have resulted in bias. Second, although the second TURBT was recommended for T1 tumors, it was performed in a few patients in this study. Third, we focused on the DWI inchworm sign in this study and did not examine other imaging methods, including an ADC map. Additional imaging methods in MRI may yield different results. Finally, BCG maintenance therapy was not administered to most patients. These limitations should be considered when interpreting the results. Further studies are required to accumulate more cases.

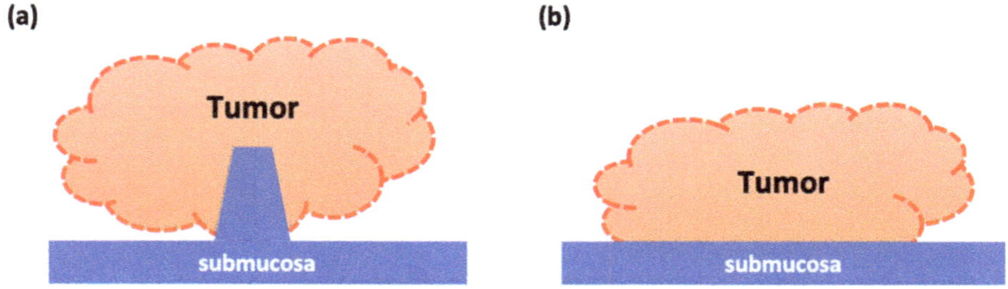

Figure 5. Schematic diagram of bladder cancer. Bladder cancer (BC) with inchworm sign has a submucosal stalk (**a**), whereas BC without inchworm sign does not (**b**). Therefore, for tumors of the same size, the surface area of the tumor protruding into the bladder lumen is larger in BC with inchworm sign (red dashed line).

5. Conclusions

The inchworm sign in BC predicted NMIBC with a high probability of 86.2%. In BC with inchworm sign, non-papillary tumors and tumors located in the bladder neck were predictors of MIBC. Although the presence of this sign indicated a high rate of NMIBC, caution should be exercised when these two factors are present. Additionally, the inchworm sign was not a prognostic factor in patients with NMIBC in this study.

Author Contributions: Conceptualization, K.I.; software, R.N. (Renato Naito) and H.Y.; formal analysis, R.N. (Ryunosuke Nakgawa); investigation, R.N. (Ryunosuke Nakagawa), S.K. (Suguru Kadomoto), H.I. and T.N.; data curation, T.N., S.K. (Shohei Kawaguchi) and K.S.; writing—original draft preparation, R.N. (Ryunosuke Nakagawa); writing—review and editing, K.I. and K.Y.; visualization, R.N. (Ryunosuke Nakagawa); supervision, K.I., Y.K. and A.M. All authors have read and agreed to the published version of the manuscript.

Funding: This research received no external funding.

Institutional Review Board Statement: The study was conducted according to the guidelines of the Declaration of Helsinki and approved by the Institutional Review Board of Kanazawa University Hospital (2021-300).

Informed Consent Statement: This study is retrospective, and informed consent was obtained in the form of opt-out posted at our facility allowed by Medical Ethics Committee of Kanazawa University. All methods were performed in accordance with relevant guidelines and regulations.

Data Availability Statement: The data presented in this study is available within the article.

Conflicts of Interest: The authors declare no conflict of interest.

Ethics Statement: All procedures performed in studies involving human participants were conducted in accordance with the ethical standards of the institutional and/or national research committee and with the 1964 Helsinki Declaration and its later amendments or comparable ethical standards.

Abbreviations

ADC (apparent diffusion coefficient); BC (bladder cancer); BCG (Bacille Calmette–Guerin); CI (confidence interval); DWI (diffusion-weighted imaging); HR (hazard ratio); MIBC (muscle invasive bladder cancer); MRI (magnetic resonance imaging); NMIBC (non-muscle invasive bladder cancer); PFS (progression-free survival); RFS (recurrence-free survival); TURBT (transurethral resection of bladder tumor).

References

1. Bray, F.; Ferlay, J.; Soerjomataram, I.; Siegel, R.L.; Torre, L.A.; Jemal, A. Global cancer statistics 2018: GLOBOCAN estimates of incidence and mortality worldwide for 36 cancers in 185 countries. *CA Cancer J. Clin.* **2018**, *68*, 394–424. [CrossRef] [PubMed]
2. Sanli, O.; Dobruch, J.; Knowles, M.A.; Burger, M.; Alemozaffar, M.; Nielsen, M.E.; Lotan, Y. Bladder cancer. *Nat. Rev. Dis. Prim.* **2017**, *3*, 17022. [CrossRef] [PubMed]
3. Witjes, J.A.; Bruins, H.M.; Cathomas, R.; Compérat, E.M.; Cowan, N.C.; Gakis, G.; Hernández, V.; Linares Espinós, E.; Lorch, A.; Neuzillet, Y.; et al. European Association of Urology Guidelines on Muscle-invasive and Metastatic Bladder Cancer: Summary of the 2020 Guidelines. *Eur. Urol.* **2021**, *79*, 82–104. [CrossRef] [PubMed]
4. Babjuk, M.; Burger, M.; Capoun, O.; Cohen, D.; Compérat, E.M.; Dominguez Escrig, J.L.; Gontero, P.; Liedberg, F.; Masson-Lecomte, A.; Mostafid, A.H.; et al. European Association of Urology Guidelines on Non-muscle-invasive Bladder Cancer (Ta, T1, and Carcinoma in Situ). *Eur. Urol.* **2022**, *81*, 75–94. [CrossRef] [PubMed]
5. Panebianco, V.; Narumi, Y.; Altun, E.; Bochner, B.H.; Efstathiou, J.A.; Hafeez, S.; Huddart, R.; Kennish, S.; Lerner, S.; Montironi, R.; et al. Multiparametric Magnetic Resonance Imaging for Bladder Cancer: Development of VI-RADS (Vesical Imaging-Reporting And Data System). *Eur. Urol.* **2018**, *74*, 294–306. [CrossRef] [PubMed]
6. Rosenkrantz, A.B.; Haghighi, M.; Horn, J.; Naik, M.; Hardie, A.D.; Somberg, M.B.; Melamed, J.; Xiao, G.Q.; Huang, W.C.; Taouli, B. Utility of quantitative MRI metrics for assessment of stage and grade of urothelial carcinoma of the bladder: Preliminary results. *AJR Am. J. Roentgenol.* **2013**, *201*, 1254–1259. [CrossRef] [PubMed]
7. Padhani, A.R.; Liu, G.; Koh, D.M.; Chenevert, T.L.; Thoeny, H.C.; Takahara, T.; Dzik-Jurasz, A.; Ross, B.D.; Van Cauteren, M.; Collins, D.; et al. Diffusion-weighted magnetic resonance imaging as a cancer biomarker: Consensus and recommendations. *Neoplasia* **2009**, *11*, 102–125. [CrossRef]
8. Yoshida, S.; Takahara, T.; Kwee, T.C.; Waseda, Y.; Kobayashi, S.; Fujii, Y. DWI as an Imaging Biomarker for Bladder Cancer. *AJR Am. J. Roentgenol.* **2017**, *208*, 1218–1228. [CrossRef]
9. El-Assmy, A.; Abou-El-Ghar, M.E.; Mosbah, A.; El-Nahas, A.R.; Refaie, H.F.; Hekal, I.A.; El-Diasty, T.; Ibrahiem el, H. Bladder tumour staging: Comparison of diffusion- and T2-weighted MR imaging. *Eur. Radiol.* **2009**, *19*, 1575–1581. [CrossRef]
10. Takeuchi, M.; Sasaki, S.; Ito, M.; Okada, S.; Takahashi, S.; Kawai, T.; Suzuki, K.; Oshima, H.; Hara, M.; Shibamoto, Y. Urinary bladder cancer: Diffusion-weighted MR imaging–accuracy for diagnosing T stage and estimating histologic grade. *Radiology* **2009**, *251*, 112–121. [CrossRef] [PubMed]
11. Saito, W.; Amanuma, M.; Tanaka, J.; Heshiki, A. Histopathological analysis of a bladder cancer stalk observed on MRI. *Magn. Reson. Imaging* **2000**, *18*, 411–415. [CrossRef] [PubMed]
12. Kobayashi, S.; Koga, F.; Yoshida, S.; Masuda, H.; Ishii, C.; Tanaka, H.; Komai, Y.; Yokoyama, M.; Saito, K.; Fujii, Y.; et al. Diagnostic performance of diffusion-weighted magnetic resonance imaging in bladder cancer: Potential utility of apparent diffusion coefficient values as a biomarker to predict clinical aggressiveness. *Eur. Radiol.* **2011**, *21*, 2178–2186. [CrossRef] [PubMed]
13. Kirkali, Z.; Chan, T.; Manoharan, M.; Algaba, F.; Busch, C.; Cheng, L.; Kiemeney, L.; Kriegmair, M.; Montironi, R.; Murphy, W.M.; et al. Bladder cancer: Epidemiology, staging and grading, and diagnosis. *Urology* **2005**, *66*, 4–34. [CrossRef] [PubMed]
14. Brooks, J.D.; Chao, W.M.; Kerr, J. Male pelvic anatomy reconstructed from the visible human data set. *J. Urol.* **1998**, *159*, 868–872. [CrossRef]
15. Li, X.M.; Yang, H.; Li, D.Q.; Zhang, P.; Ma, Q.T.; Zhai, L.D. Muscular structure at the male bladder outlet examined with successive celloidin-embedded slices. *Urology* **2015**, *85*, 629–635. [CrossRef] [PubMed]
16. Xiao, G.Q.; Rashid, H. Bladder Neck Urothelial Carcinoma: A Urinary Bladder Subsite Carcinoma With Distinct Clinicopathology. *Int. J. Surg. Pathol.* **2015**, *23*, 517–523. [CrossRef]
17. Wang, H.J.; Pui, M.H.; Guan, J.; Li, S.R.; Lin, J.H.; Pan, B.; Guo, Y. Comparison of Early Submucosal Enhancement and Tumor Stalk in Staging Bladder Urothelial Carcinoma. *AJR Am. J. Roentgenol.* **2016**, *207*, 797–803. [CrossRef]
18. Yajima, S.; Yoshida, S.; Takahara, T.; Arita, Y.; Tanaka, H.; Waseda, Y.; Yokoyama, M.; Ishioka, J.; Matsuoka, Y.; Saito, K.; et al. Usefulness of the inchworm sign on DWI for predicting pT1 bladder cancer progression. *Eur. Radiol.* **2019**, *29*, 3881–3888. [CrossRef]
19. Orsola, A.; Trias, I.; Raventós, C.X.; Español, I.; Cecchini, L.; Búcar, S.; Salinas, D.; Orsola, I. Initial high-grade T1 urothelial cell carcinoma: Feasibility and prognostic significance of lamina propria invasion microstaging (T1a/b/c) in BCG-treated and BCG-non-treated patients. *Eur. Urol.* **2005**, *48*, 231–238; discussion 238. [CrossRef]
20. Smits, G.; Schaafsma, E.; Kiemeney, L.; Caris, C.; Debruyne, F.; Witjes, J.A. Microstaging of pT1 transitional cell carcinoma of the bladder: Identification of subgroups with distinct risks of progression. *Urology* **1998**, *52*, 1009–1013; discussion 1013–1014. [CrossRef]
21. Kondylis, F.I.; Demirci, S.; Ladaga, L.; Kolm, P.; Schellhammer, P.F. Outcomes after intravesical bacillus Calmette-Guerin are not affected by substaging of high grade T1 transitional cell carcinoma. *J. Urol.* **2000**, *163*, 1120–1123. [CrossRef] [PubMed]
22. Jancke, G.; Rosell, J.; Chebil, G.; Jahnson, S. Bladder wash cytology at diagnosis of Ta-T1 bladder cancer is predictive for recurrence and progression. *Urology* **2012**, *80*, 625–631. [CrossRef] [PubMed]
23. Kiyoshima, K.; Akitake, M.; Shiota, M.; Takeuchi, A.; Takahashi, R.; Inokuchi, J.; Tatsugami, K.; Yokomizo, A.; Eto, M. Prognostic Significance of Preoperative Urine Cytology in Low-grade Non-muscle-invasive Bladder Cancer. *Anticancer Res.* **2016**, *36*, 799–802. [PubMed]

cancers

MDPI

Article

Comparison of Clinical Outcomes between Robot-Assisted Partial Nephrectomy and Cryoablation in Elderly Patients with Renal Cancer

Shohei Kawaguchi [1], Kouji Izumi [1,*], Renato Naito [1], Suguru Kadomoto [1], Hiroaki Iwamoto [1], Hiroshi Yaegashi [1], Takahiro Nohara [1], Kazuyoshi Shigehara [1], Kotaro Yoshida [2], Yoshifumi Kadono [1] and Atsushi Mizokami [1]

[1] Department of Integrative Cancer Therapy and Urology, Kanazawa University Graduate School of Medical Science, Kanazawa 920-8641, Japan
[2] Department of Radiology, Kanazawa University Graduate School of Medical Science, Kanazawa 920-8641, Japan
* Correspondence: azuizu2003@yahoo.co.jp; Tel.: +81-762652393

Simple Summary: Advances in diagnostic imaging have led to an increase in the diagnosis and treatment of small-diameter renal cell carcinomas in the elderly. Elderly patients may show impaired operative tolerance; thus, treatment should be more carefully chosen in them than in younger patients. In this study, a retrospective comparison of robot-assisted partial nephrectomy (RAPN) and percutaneous cryoablation (PCA) was conducted for small-diameter renal cell carcinomas in elderly patients. Both RAPN (with a slightly high complication rate but a low recurrence rate) and PCA (with a low complication rate but a slightly high recurrence rate) could be performed safely in elderly patients. RAPN proved to be a safe and effective method for treating small-diameter renal cell carcinomas in elderly patients, thereby being the first treatment of choice in such patients. PCA was also a safe and feasible alternative, especially in patients in whom general anesthesia poses a high risk.

Abstract: Advances in imaging technologies have increased the opportunities for treating small-diameter renal cell carcinomas (RCCs) in the elderly. This retrospective study based on real-world clinical practice compared perioperative complications, preoperative and postoperative renal function, recurrence-free survival, and overall survival in elderly patients with RCC who had undergone robot-assisted partial nephrectomy (RAPN) or percutaneous cryoablation (PCA). A total of 99 patients (aged ≥70 years), including 50 and 49 patients in the RAPN and PCA groups, respectively, were analyzed. In the entire cohort, Clavien–Dindo grade ≥3 complications occurred in only one patient who had undergone RAPN. Renal function was significantly lower in the postoperative period than in the preoperative period in both the RAPN and PCA groups. The recurrence-free survival and overall survival rates were worse in the PCA group than in the RAPN group, albeit not significantly. RAPN was considered a safe and effective method for treating RCCs in elderly patients. Moreover, although the recurrence rate was slightly higher in the PCA group than in the RAPN group, PCA was deemed to be a safe alternative, especially for treating patients in whom general anesthesia poses a high risk.

Keywords: renal cell carcinoma; robot-assisted partial nephrectomy; cryoablation; oncologic outcome; renal function

1. Introduction

Renal cell carcinoma (RCC) accounts for approximately 3% of all cancers, with an estimated peak incidence among those aged 60–70 years [1]. In recent years, the widespread use of high-resolution imaging techniques, such as computed tomography (CT) and magnetic resonance imaging (MRI), has led to an increase in the diagnosis of small, asymptomatic renal tumors [2,3]. Surgery remains the only curative treatment option for localized RCCs, and localized T1 RCCs are best managed with partial nephrectomy (PN) rather than radical nephrectomy (RN) [1]. A meta-analysis suggested that robot-assisted partial nephrectomy (RAPN), which is associated with lower estimated blood loss, shorter postoperative hospital stay, and fewer postoperative complications, might be more suitable for treating small-diameter RCCs than open nephrectomy [4].

Recently, local therapy has been recommended as an alternative approach in patients at risk for surgery, such as elderly patients and those with comorbidities [5]. While some studies suggest that RAPN and ablation therapy (AT) have similar oncological outcomes in patients with small-diameter RCCs [6], others report that the recurrence rate is significantly higher after AT than after RAPN [2,7], highlighting the need for appropriate treatment selection. Due to the increasing opportunities for treating small-diameter RCCs in the elderly, we conducted a retrospective study to compare the relationship of specific treatment approaches with clinical outcomes in real-world clinical practice.

2. Materials and Methods

This retrospective study included patients aged ≥70 years who were diagnosed with RCC and had undergone RAPN or percutaneous cryoablation (PCA) at Kanazawa University Hospital between October 2016 and December 2021. Preoperative contrast-enhanced CT and MRI were performed for staging, and tumor size and localization were evaluated using the R.E.N.A.L. score [8]. Tumors with a nephrometry score of 4, 5, or 6 points were considered to have low complexity; those with a score of 7, 8, or 9 points were deemed to have moderate complexity; and those with a score of 10, 11, or 12 points were considered to have the highest complexity [8]. In cases of renal dysfunction where the usage of a contrast medium was difficult, plain CT and MRI were used for evaluation. The indications for RAPN and PCA were determined based on the patient's general condition, complications, general anesthesia tolerance, and patient preference.

RAPN was performed using the transperitoneal or retroperitoneal approach based on the location and size of the tumor and the anatomical location of the renal vessels. Tumor resection was performed with warm ischemia using a renal artery clamp. After tumor excision, hemostasis and urinary tract repair were performed with inner sutures and parenchymal sutures were placed as needed. PCA was performed under CT guidance using the CryoHit cryoablation system (Galil Medical, Yokneam, Israel) and 17-guage cryoneedles (IceRod; Galil Medical) with local anesthesia [9]. In patients with large or hypervascular tumors at a high risk of bleeding, arterial embolization with absolute ethanol and ethiodized oil (lipiodol; Guerbet Japan, Tokyo, Japan) was performed a day before PCA. Where possible, needle biopsy was simultaneously performed with PCA to confirm the histologic type of the tumor.

Postoperative local recurrence and distant metastasis were evaluated using thoracoabdominal contrast CT. In patients who were not suitable for imaging using contrast media due to severe renal dysfunction, recurrence was evaluated using plain CT or MRI. Renal function was assessed by determining estimated glomerular filtration rates (eGFR) at 1, 3, 6, 12, and 24 months after RAPN and PCA, and postoperative eGFR preservation was calculated using the following formula: % eGFR = postoperative eGFR / preoperative eGFR × 100 [10]. The quality of RAPN was assessed using the achievement of trifecta, which was defined as a negative surgical margin, absence of postoperative complications, and warm ischemia time of ≤25 min [11].

Chi-square, Wilcoxon's signed-rank, and Mann–Whitney U tests were used to compare the features of RAPN and PCA groups. Odds ratios (ORs) with 95% confidence intervals (CIs) were used to determine the risk for a decline of ≥20% in % eGFR at postoperative year one. Multivariable logistic regression was performed to identify independent of variables. Variables with a p value of <0.1 in the univariable analysis were included in the multivariable analysis. Survival curves were measured using the Kaplan–Meier method, and differences in overall survival (OS) and recurrence-free survival (RFS) were evaluated using the log-rank test. All data analyses were performed using SPSS ver. 25.0 (SPSS, Chicago, IL, USA), and a p value of <0.05 was considered statistically significant.

3. Results

A total of 50 patients who had undergone RAPN and 49 patients who had undergone PCA at Kanazawa University Hospital were retrospectively analyzed. All analyzed patients were ≥70 years old. Table 1 shows the demographic characteristics and preoperative renal function of these 99 patients.. The median age was significantly higher in the PCA group than in the RAPN group (78 years vs. 75 years, respectively; $p = 0.010$). Although no significant differences in the incidence of hypertension, diabetes, and cardiovascular disease were observed between the two groups, cerebrovascular disease was significantly more prevalent in the PCA group than in the RAPN group ($p = 0.010$). The number of patients with a solitary kidney was significantly higher in the PCA group than in the RAPN group (8 vs. 1, $p = 0.041$). However, no significant difference in the preoperative eGFR was observed between the two groups.

Table 1. Patient characteristics and preoperative renal function.

Variable	RAPN	PCA	p Value
Patients	50	49	
Median age, years (range)	75 (70–84)	78 (70–91)	0.010
BMI, kg/m^2	23.1 ± 2.4	23.7 ± 3.8	0.324
Sex, n (%)			
Male	34 (68.0)	35 (71.4)	0.711
Female	16 (32.0)	14 (28.6)	
Hypertension, n (%)	36 (72.0)	41 (83.7)	0.069
Diabetes, n (%)	15 (30.0)	17 (34.7)	0.618
Cardiovascular disease, n (%)	7 (14.0)	5 (10.2)	0.563
Cerebrovascular disease, n (%)	3 (6.0)	12 (24.5)	0.010
Solitary kidney, n (%)	1 (2.0)	8 (16.3)	0.041
Preoperative eGFR, mL/min/1.73 m^2	65.0 ± 17.6	65.7 ± 39.1	0.334
Preoperative CKD stage			
1	3 (6.0)	9 (18.4)	
2	26 (52.0)	12 (24.5)	
3a	15 (30.0)	15 (30.6)	
3b	6 (12.0)	11 (22.4)	
4	0 (0)	1 (2.0)	
5	0 (0)	1 (2.0)	
CKD stage ≥ 3b	6 (12.0)	13 (26.5)	0.066

BMI, body mass index; CKD, chronic kidney disease; eGFR, estimated glomerular filtration rate; PCA, percutaneous cryoablation; RAPN, robot-assisted partial nephrectomy.

Table 2 presents the reasons for choosing PCA in the study cohort. Ten patients were unable to tolerate general anesthesia and harbored absolute contraindications for RAPN. Seventeen patients harbored relative contraindications for RAPN due to a solitary kidney, previous surgery, renal vascular abnormalities, or difficulty in intraoperative tumor identification. Most patients had comorbidities, and PCA was performed in only three patients without comorbidities based on patient preference.

The tumor features are shown in Table 3. In brief, the maximum tumor diameter was 2.7 ± 1.2 cm in the RAPN group and 2.4 ± 0.8 cm in the PCA group, with no significant difference between the two groups. Most of the patients in both the groups had clinical Ta RCC, and the R.E.N.A.L. scores were low or moderate in most patients.

Table 2. Reasons for choosing PCA.

Reasons	Details	$n = 49$
Absolute contraindications for RAPN (general anesthesia not available)		
Respiratory diseases	Interstitial pneumonia	3
	Chronic obstructive pulmonary disease	2
	Pyothorax	1
Cardiovascular diseases	Chronic heart failure	2
	Cardiomyopathy	1
	Valvular disease	1
Relative contraindications for RAPN		
Solitary kidney		8
History of previous surgery	Major abdominal surgery	2
	Partial nephrectomy	2
Renal vascular abnormality	Renal artery aneurysm	1
	Renal artery stenosis	1
Difficulty in tumor identification	Polycystic kidney disease	2
	Abnormal renal morphology	1
Patient preference or physician recommendation		
Under treatment for other cancers	Castration-resistant prostate cancer	3
	Hepatocellular carcinoma	2
	Chronic myelogenous leukemia	1
Bilateral or multiple renal tumor	Bilateral	3
	Multiple	1
Extreme age (>85 years old)		4
Patients with comorbidities	Ischemic heart disease	2
	Cerebrovascular disease	2
	Low respiratory function after lung cancer surgery	1
Patients without comorbidities		3

PCA, percutaneous cryoablation; RAPN, robot-assisted partial nephrectomy.

The surgical margins were positive in 2 (4.0%) patients, and trifecta was achieved in 36 (72.0%) patients. In the entire study cohort, Clavien–Dindo grade ≥3 complications were observed in only one patient (grade 3a pneumothorax) who had undergone RAPN. The mean follow-up period was 24.3 (2–60) months and 20.1 (2–60) months for the RAPN and PCA groups, respectively.

In the RAPN group, the preoperative mean eGFR was 65.0 ± 17.6 mL/min/1.73 m^2 and the postoperative eGFR was significantly lower than the preoperative eGFR at all timepoints. In particular, the postoperative eGFRs at 1, 3, 6, 12, and 24 months were 62.4 ± 19.6 (p = 0.021), 60.5 ± 18.5 (p = 0.002), 59.5 ± 17.9 (p <0.001), 58.8 ± 17.7 (p <0.001), and 64.1 ± 20.1 (p = 0.001) mL/min/1.73 m^2, respectively. In the PCA group, the preoperative mean eGFR was 65.7 ± 39.1 mL/min/1.73 m^2 and the postoperative eGFR was significantly lower than the preoperative eGFR at all timepoints. In particular, the postoperative eGFRs at 1, 3, 6, 12, and 24 months were 55.9 ± 22.2 (p <0.001), 54.9 ± 22.5 (p <0.001), 51.0 ± 17.9 (p <0.001), 51.6 ± 20.7 (p <0.001), and 46.4 ± 17.5 (p = 0.001) mL/min/1.73 m^2, respectively.

The changes in % eGFR are shown in Figure 1. Although many patients in the two groups had preserved renal function in the early post-treatment period, the percentage of patients with a % eGFR of <90% increased over time. The univariableanalysis performed to determine factors associated with a >20% reduction in % eGFR at postoperative year 1 showed no significant associations with age, sex, body mass index, hypertension, diabetes mellitus, treatment type (RAPN vs. PCA), and preoperative stage 3a or higher chronic kidney disease (CKD) (Table 4). The univariable and multivariable analyses indicated that an R.E.N.A.L score ≥7 points was a risk factor for >20% reduction in % eGFR at postoperative year 1.

Table 3. Tumor features in patients who had undergone RAPN or PCA.

Variable	RAPN	PCA	*p* Value
Maximum tumor diameter, cm	2.7 ± 1.2	2.4 ± 0.8	0.204
Laterality, *n* (%)			
Left	27 (54.0)	29 (59.2)	
Right	23 (46.0)	20 (40.8)	
Clinical T stage			
T1a	42 (84.0)	46 (93.9)	
T1b	8 (16.0)	1 (4.0)	
T3a	0 (0)	2 (4.1)	
R.E.N.A.L. score			
Low (4–6)	29 (59.2)	32 (65.3)	
Moderate (7–9)	20 (40.0)	17 (34.7)	
Highest (10–12)	1 (2.0)	0 (0)	
Pathologic T stage			
T1a	39 (78.0)		
T1b	5 (10.0)		
T3a	4 (8.0)		
Benign	2 (4.0)		
Histologic subtype			
Clear cell	35 (50.0)	38 (77.6)	
Papillary	6 (12.0)	1 (2.0)	
Chromophobe	3 (6.0)	1 (2.0)	
Benign	2 (4.0)	2 (4.1)	
Others	4 (8.0)	0 (0)	
Nondiagnostic	0 (0)	7 (14.3)	

PCA, percutaneous cryoablation; RAPN, robot-assisted partial nephrectomy.

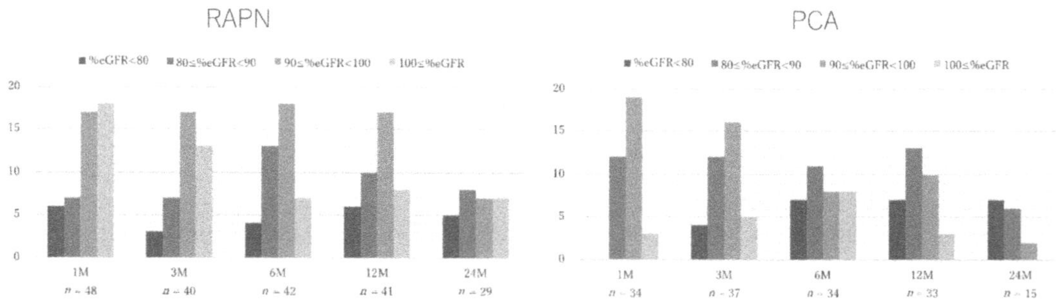

Figure 1. Changes in renal function. Changes in renal function declined in the postoperative period compared with the preoperative period in patients who had undergone robotic-assisted partial nephrectomy (RAPN) and percutaneous cryoablation (PCA). eGFR, estimated glomerular filtration rate.

Figure 2 compares the RFS and OS of the patients in the RAPN and PCA groups, excluding two cases, each with benign histology. In brief, the log-rank test revealed that the OS and RFS were slightly worse in the PCA group than in the RAPN group, albeit not significantly (OS, p = 0.160; RFS, p = 0.105). Fournier's gangrene was the cause of death in the RAPN group, whereas prostate cancer, interstitial pneumonia, myocardial infarction, and multiple organ failure were the causes of death in the PCA group. There were no deaths due to RCC in either group.

Table 4. Results of univariable and multivariable logistic regression analyses for factors associated with the risk of % eGFR <80% at postoperative year 1.

Factor	Patients with %eGFR <80% at Postoperative Year 1			
	Univariable Logistic Regression		Multivariable Logistic Regression	
	p Value	OR (95% CI)	*p* Value	OR (95% CI)
Age (≥ 78 years)	0.782	1.190 (0.346–4.097)		
Sex, female	0.077	3.020 (0.886–10.286)	0.079	3.270 (0.873–12.244)
BMI (≥25 kg/m^2)	0.276	0.463 (0.115–1.854)		
Hypertension	0.478	1.793 (0.357–9.021)		
Diabetes mellitus	0.127	2.579 (0.763–8.715)		
Treatment, RAPN	0.462	0.637 (0.191–2.120)		
Preoperative CKD stage (≥3a)	0.625	1.358 (0.399–4.624)		
R.E.N.A.L. score (≥moderate)	0.008	5.824 (1.581–21.454)	0.008	6.136 (1.596–23.585)

BMI, body mass index; CI, confidence interval; CKD, chronic kidney disease; eGFR, estimated glomerular filtration rate; OR, odds ratio; RAPN, robot-assisted partial nephrectomy.

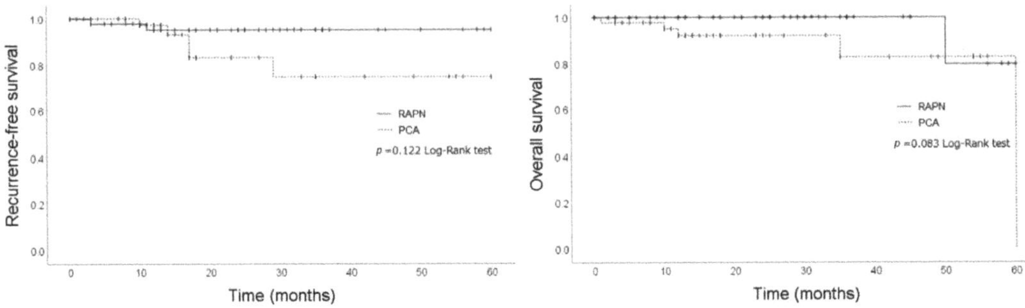

Figure 2. Recurrence-free survival and overall survival. Comparison of recurrence-free survival and overall survival between patients who had undergone robot-assisted partial nephrectomy (RAPN) and those who had undergone percutaneous cryoablation (PCA).

4. Discussion

Cancer-specific survival rates are comparable between PN and RN for localized RCCs, and PN achieves better preservation of renal function than RN, thereby reducing the incidence of metabolic and cardiovascular disorders. Therefore, the best treatment option for localized T1 RCC is PN rather than RN [1]. RAPN is associated with lower blood loss, fewer transfusions and postoperative complications, and lower eGFR decline than PN [12]. In addition, RAPN has been shown to achieve a significantly shorter warm ischemic time and a higher trifecta attainment rate than laparoscopic PN (LPN), indicating its possible advantage in the preservation of renal function [13,14]. Although a high hospitalization cost is a disadvantage, RAPN is superior than other treatment methods, even in frail patients, owing to fewer complications associated with it and shorter hospital stays [15].

Although PN is an appropriate treatment option for localized RCCs as it preserves renal function and has good oncological outcomes, it requires general anesthesia and may not be a feasible option depending on the patient's general condition, such as impaired cardiac or respiratory function. PCA is a minimally invasive procedure that does not require general anesthesia and can be performed in patients who cannot tolerate general anesthesia. In the present study, 10 of the 49 patients (20.4%) who had undergone PCA could not tolerate general anesthesia. In addition, the patients in the PCA group were significantly older and had a higher rate of cerebrovascular diseases than those in the RAPN group; however, the rates of hypertension, diabetes, and cardiovascular diseases were not significantly different between the two groups. PCA might have been preferred over RAPN due to decreased daily living activities and poor general condition as a result of the advanced age and cerebrovascular disease history.

Studies have reported that the rate of complications is slightly higher for RAPN and LPN than for PCA (Clavien–Dindo grade ≥3 complication rate: 2.6% in RAPN vs. 2.1% in PCA; 3.3% in LPN vs. 1.1% PCA), although the differences were not statistically significant [6,10]. A higher incidence of acute kidney injury with PN than with AT, including radiofrequency ablation and PCA, has also been reported [7]. In the present study, the higher number of patients with a solitary kidney in the PCA group was considered a rational reason for the chosen approach, given the risk of acute kidney injury. There was only one patient with a Clavien–Dindo grade ≥3 complication in the RAPN group, suggesting that RAPN can be safely performed in patients aged ≥70 years. However, PCA may be a safer approach than RAPN because none of the patients who had undergone PCA developed Clavien–Dindo grade ≥3 complications in the present study.

However, a previous study reporting on the 5-year follow-up data of minimally invasive PN (LPN or RAPN) and AT revealed a significantly higher local recurrence rate in the AT group than in the PN group (21.2% vs. 4.7%) [7]. A meta-analysis also reported significantly worse local RFS after AT [16]. In the present study, the RFS was slightly worse in the PCA group than in the RAPN group, albeit not significantly. Local recurrence requires other treatment approaches, such as surgery and AT, and strict follow-up with imaging studies is considered necessary, especially after PCA. RAPN may be a good option for the elderly, considering the low risk of recurrence, consequent re-treatment.

A previous study demonstrated that RAPN is associated with a higher trifecta achievement rate and less deterioration in postoperative renal function compared with LPN [13]. Another study reported that the reduction in eGFR after PCA was not significant [17]. Glomerular filtration rate has been reported to decline with age in elderly patients, even in healthy individuals without any underlying disease [18]. Furthermore, elderly patients have several comorbidities, and the decline in glomerular filtration rate in the elderly is largely due to the presence of comorbidities in addition to normal aging [19]. In the present study, our assessment regarding the preservation of renal function revealed a significant decrease in eGFR in the postoperative period compared with the preoperative period in both the RAPN and PCA groups. The participants in the present study were ≥70 years, and there is a possibility that the observed decline in renal function was due to the high prevalence of comorbidities, such as hypertension and diabetes mellitus. In a previous study, multivariable analysis revealed that a higher R.E.N.A.L score was a significant factor of ≥10% decrease in eGFR at 6 months after RAPN and PCA [6]. In the present study, both the univariable and multivariable analyses revealed that an R.E.N.A.L score of ≥7 was significantly associated with a decline of ≥20% in %eGFR at 1 year after treatment. Therefore, a high R.E.N.A.L score might be a predictor of decreased postoperative renal function.

In patients undergoing PN, initial tumor pathological characteristics and subsequent radiologic imaging results are used to determine treatment success, whereas in patients undergoing AT, radiologic evaluation is used to determine treatment success [20]. Although contrast-enhanced CT or contrast-enhanced MRI is often used to evaluate recurrence after treatment, the use of contrast material may be difficult in patients with impaired renal function due to concerns about contrast-induced nephropathy and nephrogenic systemic fibrosis [21]. The sensitivity of plain CT and plain MRI in detecting locally recurrent lesions is low, which is a concern that should be considered, especially after AT in patients with a high local recurrence rate. The feasibility of follow-up imaging with 111In-girentuximab single-photon emission CT has been reported after PCA for RCC; this approach may improve early detection of residual or recurrent disease and may also be applied in patients with inadequate renal function [22].

The main limitations of the present study were its retrospective study design and small sample size. This study used real-world data, with significantly more patients with T1b tumors in the RAPN group and significantly more patients with a solitary kidney in the PCA group. This difference may have impacted oncological outcomes and post-treatment renal function. Moreover, the follow-up period was short, and only a few patients in the PCA group could be evaluated for renal function at 2 years. Patients with stage 3b or higher CKD were also included, and follow-up imaging might not have accurately assessed recurrence due to the need to reduce or not use contrast media. Because of the lack of clear criteria for treatment selection and significant differences in baseline age, the oncological outcomes and changes in renal function could not be accurately assessed. In addition, a no-treatment follow-up is possible with a longer doubling time in patients with RCC who are older and have more comorbidities; however, this study did not investigate patients on a no-treatment follow-up.

5. Conclusions

In elderly patients aged ≥70 years diagnosed with RCC, RAPN was a safe and effective treatment approach with a high nonrecurrence rate. Despite a slightly higher recurrence rate than RAPN, PCA was deemed to be a safe and feasible alternative, especially in patients in whom general anesthesia poses a high risk.

Author Contributions: Conceptualization, K.I. and S.K. (Shohei Kawaguchi); Methodology, S.K. (Shohei Kawaguchi); Investigation, S.K. (Shohei Kawaguchi), T.N. and K.S.; Data Curation, S.K. (Shohei Kawaguchi), K.I., R.N., S.K. (Suguru Kadomoto), H.I., H.Y., T.N., K.S., K.Y., Y.K. and A.M.; Writing—Original Draft Preparation, S.K. (Shohei Kawaguchi); Writing—Review and Editing, S.K. (Shohei Kawaguchi), K.Y. and K.I.; Supervision, K.I. and Y.K.; Project Administration, A.M. All authors have read and agreed to the published version of the manuscript.

Funding: This research received no external funding.

Institutional Review Board Statement: The study was conducted according to the guidelines of the Declaration of Helsinki, and approved by the Institutional Review Board of Kanazawa University Hospital (approval no: 113959-1; date of approval: 20 April 2022).

Informed Consent Statement: Patient consent was obtained through the opt-out option on the website.

Data Availability Statement: The data presented in this study is available within the article.

Conflicts of Interest: There are no financial or other relations that could lead to a conflict of interest regarding this study.

References

1. Ljungberg, B.; Albiges, L.; Abu-Ghanem, Y.; Bedke, J.; Capitanio, U.; Dabestani, S.; Fernández-Pello, S.; Giles, R.H.; Hofmann, F.; Hora, M.; et al. European association of urology guidelines on renal cell carcinoma: The 2022 update. *Eur. Urol.* **2022**, *82*, 399–410. [CrossRef] [PubMed]
2. Fraisse, G.; Colleter, L.; Peyronnet, B.; Khene, Z.E.; Mandoorah, Q.; Soorojebally, Y.; Bourgi, A.; De La Taille, A.; Roupret, M.; De Kerviler, E.; et al. Peri-operative and local control outcomes of robot-assisted partial nephrectomy vs percutaneous cryoablation for renal masses: Comparison after matching on radiological stage and renal score. *BJU Int.* **2019**, *123*, 632–638. [CrossRef] [PubMed]
3. Makino, T.; Izumi, K.; Iwamoto, H.; Kadomoto, S.; Naito, R.; Yaegashi, H.; Shigehara, K.; Kadono, Y.; Mizokami, A. The impact of hypertension on the clinicopathological outcome and progression of renal cell carcinoma. *Anticancer Res.* **2020**, *40*, 4087–4093. [CrossRef]
4. Ni, Y.; Yang, X. A systematic review and meta-analysis of comparison of outcomes of robot-assisted versus open partial nephrectomy in clinical t1 renal cell carcinoma patients. *Urol. Int.* **2022**, *106*, 757–767. [CrossRef] [PubMed]
5. Salagierski, M.; Wojciechowska, A.; Zając, K.; Klatte, T.; Thompson, R.H.; Cadeddu, J.A.; Kaouk, J.; Autorino, R.; Ahrar, K.; Capitanio, U. The role of ablation and minimally invasive techniques in the management of small renal masses. *Eur. Urol. Oncol.* **2018**, *1*, 395–402. [CrossRef] [PubMed]
6. Uemura, T.; Kato, T.; Nagahara, A.; Kawashima, A.; Hatano, K.; Ujike, T.; Ono, Y.; Higashihara, H.; Fujita, K.; Fukuhara, S.; et al. Therapeutic and clinical outcomes of robot-assisted partial nephrectomy versus cryoablation for t1 renal cell carcinoma. *In Vivo* **2021**, *35*, 1573–1579. [CrossRef]
7. Bianchi, L.; Chessa, F.; Piazza, P.; Ercolino, A.; Mottaran, A.; Recenti, D.; Serra, C.; Gaudiano, C.; Cappelli, A.; Modestino, F.; et al. Percutaneous ablation or minimally invasive partial nephrectomy for ct1a renal masses? A propensity score-matched analysis. *Int. J. Urol.* **2022**, *29*, 222–228. [CrossRef]
8. Kutikov, A.; Uzzo, R.G. The R.E.N.A.L. Nephrometry score: A comprehensive standardized system for quantitating renal tumor size, location and depth. *J. Urol.* **2009**, *182*, 844–853. [CrossRef]

9. Michimoto, K.; Shimizu, K.; Kameoka, Y.; Sadaoka, S.; Miki, J.; Kishimoto, K. Transcatheter arterial embolization with a mixtur of absolute ethanol and iodized oil for poorly visualized endophytic renal masses prior to ct-guided percutaneous cryoablatio *Cardiovasc. Interv. Radiol.* **2016**, *39*, 1589–1594. [CrossRef]
10. Yanagisawa, T.; Miki, J.; Shimizu, K.; Fukuokaya, W.; Urabe, F.; Mori, K.; Sasaki, H.; Kimura, T.; Miki, K.; Egawa, S. Functiona and oncological outcome of percutaneous cryoablation versus laparoscopic partial nephrectomy for clinical t1 renal tumors: A propensity score-matched analysis. *Urol. Oncol.* **2020**, *38*, 938.e1–938.e7. [CrossRef]
11. Hung, A.J.; Cai, J.; Simmons, M.N.; Gill, I.S. "Trifecta" in partial nephrectomy. *J. Urol.* **2013**, *189*, 36–42. [CrossRef] [PubMed]
12. Tsai, S.H.; Tseng, P.T.; Sherer, B.A.; Lai, Y.C.; Lin, P.Y.; Wu, C.K.; Stoller, M.L. Open versus robotic partial nephrectomy: Systemati review and meta-analysis of contemporary studies. *Int. J. Med. Robot.* **2019**, *15*, e1963. [CrossRef] [PubMed]
13. Kawase, K.; Enomoto, T.; Kawase, M.; Takai, M.; Kato, D.; Fujimoto, S.; Iinuma, K.; Nakane, K.; Kato, S.; Hagiwara, N.; et al. Th impact of postoperative renal function recovery after laparoscopic and robot-assisted partial nephrectomy in patients with rena cell carcinoma. *Medicina* **2022**, *58*, 485. [CrossRef] [PubMed]
14. Ohba, K.; Matsuo, T.; Mitsunari, K.; Nakamura, Y.; Nakanishi, H.; Mochizuki, Y.; Miyata, Y. Preservation of split renal functio after laparoscopic and robot-assisted partial nephrectomy. *Anticancer Res.* **2022**, *42*, 3055–3060. [CrossRef] [PubMed]
15. Rosiello, G.; Palumbo, C.; Deuker, M.; Stolzenbach, L.F.; Martin, T.; Tian, Z.; Larcher, A.; Capitanio, U.; Montorsi, F.; Shariat, S.F et al. Partial nephrectomy in frail patients: Benefits of robot-assisted surgery. *Surg. Oncol.* **2021**, *38*, 101588. [CrossRef] [PubMed
16. Chan, V.W.; Abul, A.; Osman, F.H.; Ng, H.H.; Wang, K.; Yuan, Y.; Cartledge, J.; Wah, T.M. Ablative therapies versus partia nephrectomy for small renal masses—A systematic review and meta-analysis. *Int. J. Surg.* **2022**, *97*, 106194. [CrossRef]
17. Zhou, W.; Herwald, S.E.; McCarthy, C.; Uppot, R.N.; Arellano, R.S. Radiofrequency ablation, cryoablation, and microwave ablation for t1a renal cell carcinoma: A comparative evaluation of therapeutic and renal function outcomes. *J. Vasc. Interv. Radiol* **2019**, *30*, 1035–1042. [CrossRef]
18. Eriksen, B.O.; Palsson, R.; Ebert, N.; Melsom, T.; van der Giet, M.; Gudnason, V.; Indridason, O.S.; Inker, L.A.; Jenssen, T.G. Levey, A.S.; et al. Gfr in healthy aging: An individual participant data meta-analysis of iohexol clearance in european population based cohorts. *J. Am. Soc. Nephrol.* **2020**, *31*, 1602–1615. [CrossRef]
19. Abdulkader, R.; Burdmann, E.A.; Lebrão, M.L.; Duarte, Y.A.O.; Zanetta, D.M.T. Aging and decreased glomerular filtration rate An elderly population-based study. *PLoS ONE* **2017**, *12*, e0189935. [CrossRef]
20. Ortiz-Alvarado, O.; Anderson, J.K. The role of radiologic imaging and biopsy in renal tumor ablation. *World J. Urol.* **2010**, *28*, 551–557. [CrossRef]
21. Gobara, H.; Nakatsuka, A.; Shimizu, K.; Yamanaka, T.; Matsui, Y.; Iguchi, T.; Hiraki, T.; Yamakado, K. Cryoablation of renal cell carcinoma for patients with stage 4 or 5 non-dialysis chronic kidney disease. *Jpn. J. Radiol.* **2019**, *37*, 481–486. [CrossRef] [PubMed]
22. Van Oostenbrugge, T.J.; Langenhuijsen, J.F.; Oosterwijk, E.; Boerman, O.C.; Jenniskens, S.F.; Oyen, W.J.G.; Fütterer, J.J.; Mulders, P.F.A. Follow-up imaging after cryoablation of clear cell renal cell carcinoma is feasible using single photon emission computed tomography with (111)in-girentuximab. *Eur. J. Nucl. Med. Mol. Imaging* **2020**, *47*, 1864–1870. [CrossRef] [PubMed]

cancers

Article

Sutureless Purely Off-Clamp Robot-Assisted Partial Nephrectomy: Avoiding Renorrhaphy Does Not Jeopardize Surgical and Functional Outcomes

Aldo Brassetti [1,*], Leonardo Misuraca [1], Umberto Anceschi [1], Alfredo Maria Bove [1], Manuela Costantini [1], Maria Consiglia Ferriero [1], Salvatore Guaglianone [1], Riccardo Mastroianni [1], Giulia Torregiani [2], Marco Covotta [2], Gabriele Tuderti [1] and Giuseppe Simone [1]

1 Department of Urology, IRCCS "Regina Elena" National Cancer Institute, 00144 Rome, Italy
2 Department of Anesthesiology, IRCCS "Regina Elena" National Cancer Institute, 00144 Rome, Italy
* Correspondence: aldo.brassetti@gmail.com; Tel.: +39-0652666772

Simple Summary: Suturing the kidney after tumor excision can be omitted most of the time, without increasing the risks of complications or jeopardizing renal function.

Abstract: To compare outcomes of sutureless (SL) vs. renorrhaphy (RR) off-clamp robotic partial nephrectomy (ocRPN), we retrospectively analyzed procedures performed at our center, from January 2017 to April 2021, for cT1-2N0M0 renal masses. All the patients with a minimum follow-up < 1 month were excluded from the analysis. The trifecta rate defined surgical quality. Any worsening from chronic kidney disease (CKD) I-II to ≧ IIIa (from IIIa to ≧ IIIb, and from IIIb to ≧ IV) was considered as significant stage migration (sCKDsm). A 1:1 propensity score-matched (PSM) analysis minimized baseline imbalances between SL and RR cohorts in terms of age, gender, ASA score, baseline estimated glomerular filtration rate (eGFR), tumor size, and RENAL score. Logistic regression analyses identified predictors of trifecta achievement. Kaplan–Meier (KM) analysis assessed the impact of RR on significant chronic kidney disease sCKDsm-free survival (SMFS), while Cox regression analyses identified its predictors. Overall, 531 patients were included, with a median tumor size of 3.5 cm (IQR: 2.7–5); 70 (13%) presented with a cT2 mass. An SL approach was pursued in 180 cases, but 10 needed conversion to RR. After PSM analysis, patients receiving SL showed a higher trifecta rate (94% vs. 84%; $p = 0.007$). SMFS probabilities were comparable at KM analysis (log-rank = 0.69). Age (OR: 0.97; 95%CI: 0.95–0.99; $p = 0.01$), a RENAL score ≧ 10 (OR: 0.29; 95%CI: 0.15–0.57; $p < 0.001$), and RR (OR: 0.34; 95%CI: 0.17–0.67; $p = 0.002$) were independent predictors of trifecta achievement. Age (OR: 1.04; 95%CI: 1.003–1.07; $p = 0.03$) and baseline eGFR (OR: 0.99; 95%CI: 0.97–0.99; $p = 0.05$) independently predicted sCKDsm. Compared to RR, our experience seems to show that the SL approach significantly increased the probabilities of achieving the trifecta in the observed group of cases.

Keywords: partial nephrectomy; renorrhaphy; sutureless; renal function; renal cancer

1. Introduction

Over the last decades, the improvement and spread of nephron-sparing surgery (NSS) techniques, together with the increasing trend in the use of robot-assisted partial nephrectomy (RAPN) for the treatment of renal masses, led to the adoption of radical nephrectomy for cT1 renal masses to less than 10%, especially in high volume centers [1].

However, despite the efforts to preserve long-term renal function and minimize the risk of acute kidney injury, up to 30% of patients with normal preoperative kidney function may experience a decline in estimated glomerular filtration rate (eGFR) to <60 mL/min/1.73 m^2, and up to 10% may have a 50% reduction in renal function after surgery [2]. Thus, the search for innovative techniques to improve long-term functional outcomes after nephron-sparing surgery (NSS) is ongoing.

There is grounded evidence that every minute of warm ischemia significantly affects short- and long-term renal function [3]. Selective renal artery clamping [4], early unclamping [5], and off-clamp surgery [6] may help reduce the risk of postoperative renal function impairment. According to limited data, renorrhaphy (RR) may adversely affect functional outcomes, leading to ischemic necrosis of the stitched parenchyma [7,8] and potentially causing pseudoaneurysms and arteriovenous fistulas [9].

Since the pioneering era of minimally invasive PN, we aimed at minimizing ischemia "whenever feasible"; in 2012, we reported the feasibility and safety of *sutureless* [SL] laparoscopic PN for small exophytic renal tumors [10]. This experience shed light on the possibility of simplifying surgical procedures (in selected cases) and optimizing functional outcomes without jeopardizing oncologic results. However, the selection bias of that study limited the employment of the SL approach in intermediate/high nephrometry score renal tumors. In the last decade, we have witnessed the wide spreading of robotic platforms, and RAPN has overcome the laparoscopic approach for the treatment of all renal tumors. In this scenario, we developed a purely off-clamp SL robotic technique that completely avoids both hilar clamping and RR, based on the selective control of feeding arteries during tumor enucleation and the monopolar cauterization of the parenchymal breach to achieve hemostasis. In the present paper, we compare surgical and functional outcomes of patients who underwent purely off-clamp RAPN (ocRAPN), with or without RR, at our institution.

2. Materials and Methods

2.1. Patients and Dataset

After review board approval, our prospectively maintained database was queried for patients who underwent ocRAPN for organ-confined (cT1-2N0M0) renal tumors, from January 2017 onwards. Starting from January 2020, all the NSSs were performed with an SL approach; intraoperative conversion to RR was only deemed necessary in case of renal calyx violation with an obvious urinary leak and/or insufficient hemostasis at the first attempt of coagulation of the parenchymal breach.

The following data were extracted:

1. Age, gender, and race;
2. Baseline American Society of Anesthesiologists (ASA) score;
3. Tumor side, clinical size, and surgical complexity (defined according to the R.E.N.A.L. score) [11];
4. Hemostatic technique and eventual conversions from SL to RR;
5. Serum creatinine levels assessed at baseline, at discharge, and 3, 6, and 12 months after surgery. For each timepoint, eGFR was calculated by means of the Chronic Kidney Disease Epidemiology Collaboration formula [12] and the National Kidney Foundation (NKF); chronic kidney disease (CKD) stages were defined accordingly [13]. Based on the NKF recommendations, a >30% reduction in the postoperative eGFR was considered as a "significant renal function deterioration" (sRFD), while any worsening from stages I-II to $\geqq$ IIIa (from IIIa to $\geqq$ IIIb, and from IIIb to $\geqq$ IV) was defined as "significant CKD stage migration" (sCKDsm) [14,15];
6. Postoperative complications (stratified according to the Clavien–Dindo (CD) classification system [16]) and length of hospital stay (LOS);
7. Perioperative outcomes combined into our previously published trifecta (negative surgical margins, no CD $\geqq$ 3 complications, and no sRFD) to assess surgical quality [14].
8. Final histology;
9. Functional outcomes at last available follow-up.

2.2. *Perioperative Care and Surgical Technique*

All the procedures were performed by one single experienced robotic surgeon (G.S.). The surgical technique for conventional ocRPN with RR was previously described [17], and its principles remained unchanged, except for the postenucleation hemostasis. A single dose of cefazolin was given intravenously, 20 min before the skin incision. A transurethral urinary catheter was inserted, and the patient was placed in an extended flank position. The camera port was placed on the pararectal line, at the level of the umbilicus, and two other robotic cannulas were placed along the midclavicular and anterior axillary line, respectively. Two laparoscopic 12 mm trocars for the table-side assistant were positioned midway between the camera and each robotic port, thus creating a U-shape disposition focused on the tumor. The *daVinci Xi*™ surgical platform (Intuitive Surgical, Sunnyvale, CA, USA), equipped with the *ERBE VIO dV 2.0*™ energy generator, was docked from the patient's back. Three robotic instruments were used: a 30° 3DHD endoscope, monopolar curved scissors, and *ProGrasp*™ forceps (Intuitive Surgical). The two 12 mm assistant ports allowed the introduction of two suction-irrigation devices. The surgery was always carried out through a three-arm transperitoneal approach. The colon was medialized, and the Gerota's fascia was opened, directly chasing the tumor. Dissection of the renal hilum was not attempted, as in no case were the vessels clamped. In fact, an hilum-sparing approach helps reduce surgical times while limiting accidental vascular injuries and, ultimately, intraoperative blood loss [18]. Straight access to the neoplasm was always pursued; thus, an extensive mobilization of the kidney was only required in the case of posterior tumors. Once the renal mass was identified, its margins were marked with cautery, intra-abdominal pressure was temporarily risen from 12 to 20 mmHg, and enucleation was begun. This step was carried out with blunt dissection, following an almost avascular plane, while the two suction-irrigation devices helped maintain a clear surgical field, combining irrigation and suction. The feeding arteries identified during the enucleation were progressively controlled with monopolar coagulation, but complete hemostasis was only pursued once the tumor was excised; then, monopolar cautery (*SwiftCOAG*™ waveform, effect 8, with an 80 W limit) was extensively applied to the resection bed, under an appropriate dripping of saline solution, while blood was aspirated. Once a firm uniform eschar covered the entire resection bed and no bleeders were observed, the pneumoperitoneum was lowered down to 5 mmHg, and hemostasis was checked for 5 min. Topical hemostatic agents were never used to improve bleeding control. An EndoCatch™ device was used to retrieve the specimen.

Postoperative pain control was achieved using intravenous nonopioid analgesics, with a gradual transition to oral painkillers. On postoperative day (POD) 1, both the abdominal drain and urethral catheter were usually removed, oral intake was initiated, and patients were encouraged to ambulate. The drain was left in place when the 24 h output was >100 mL.

2.3. Study Objective

The aim of the present study was to present our novel SL surgical technique and report our single-center experience of 175 cases, retrospectively comparing outcomes with those of the conventional ocRAPN with RR.

2.4. Statistical Analysis

The study population was split into 2 groups according to hemostasis technique (RR vs. SL). After excluding 37 patients (7%) who underwent further renal surgeries because of bilateral tumors or renal stones, a 1:1 propensity score-matched (PSM) analysis was used to minimize imbalances between the two cohorts in variables potentially affecting outcomes (age, gender, ASA score, baseline eGFR, and RENAL score); the model was set to provide a standardized mean difference $\leqslant$10% between covariates. Frequencies and proportions were used to report categorical variables, which were compared by means of the χ^2 test. Continuous variables were presented as median and interquartile ranges (IQRs) and were compared using either the Mann–Whitney U test or Kruskal–Wallis one-way analysis based on their normal or not-normal distribution, respectively (the normality of the distribution of variables was tested by the Kolmogorov–Smirnov test). Kaplan–Meier (KM) analysis and a log-rank test assessed the impact of surgical technique on sCKDsm-free survival (SMFS), while Cox regression analyses identified its predictors. Univariable and multivariable logistic regression analyses were performed to identify predictors of trifecta nonachievement and sRFI. The significance threshold was set at <0.05. Statistical analysis was performed using the Statistical Package for Social Science v. 25.0 (IBM, Somers, NY, USA).

3. Results

Out of 548 cases of ocRAPN, 15 were lost to follow-up and excluded from the analysis. Among the remaining 533 patients, 185 were offered an SL approach, but 10 (5%) required conversion to RR due to intraoperative suspicion of urinary calyx injury (n = 8) or uncontrollable bleeding (n = 2); therefore, they were ultimately allocated to the RR group (Supplementary Materials Table S1).

Overall, the median age of our study population was 62 years (IQR: 54–71), and the average tumor size was 3.5 cm (IQR: 2.7–5); the observed trifecta rate was 86% (Table 1). Compared to those in the RR group (n = 358), patients from the SL cohort were significantly older (64 years vs. 61 years; p = 0.04) and less frequently harbored highly complex neoplasms (RENAL score ≥ 10) (17% vs. 23%; p = 0.005) (Table 1). Major complications (2% vs. 5%; p = 0.06) and transfusion (3% vs. 5%; p = 0.40) rates were not statistically different in the two groups. Overall, five (1%) urinary fistulas at the level of the parenchymal breach were observed after surgery (three and two in the SL and RR groups, respectively; p = 0.18), and they all healed spontaneously after ureteral stent placement. Selective embolization under general anesthesia was required 16 times overall because of post-RAPN bleeding.

Table 1. Patients' characteristics and outcomes after ocRPN.

	Overall n **= 533**	**SL** n **= 175 (33%)**	**RR** n **= 358 (67%)**	p	**PSM SL** n **= 80**	**PSM RR** n **= 80**	p
Age, years	62 (54–71)	64 (55–72)	61 (52–70)	0.04	64 (56–73)	64 (55–73)	0.84
Male gender, n (%)	333 (62%)	108 (62%)	225 (63%)	0.79	51 (64%)	53 (66%)	0.74
ASA ≧ 3, n (%)	124 (23%)	32 (18%)	92 (26%)	0.06	13 (16%)	21 (26%)	0.12
Baseline eGFR, ml/min	81.8 (69.4–95.7)	82.1 (68.3–97.2)	81.7 (69.7–94.2)	0.59	79 (66.9–95.1)	78.1 (69.5–93.5)	0.86
Baseline CKD stage							
1–2	466 (87%)	155 (88%)	311 (87%)	0.76	71 (89%)	70 (88%)	0.74
3A–3B	59 (11%)	17 (10%)	42 (12%)		7 (9%)	9 (11%)	
4–5	8 (2%)	3 (2%)	5 (1%)		2 (2%)	1 (1%)	
Tumor size, cm	3.5 (2.5–5)	3 (2.5–5)	4 (3–5)	0.16	3 (2.5–4.5)	3.5 (2.5–5)	0.70
cT2, n (%)	70 (13%)	20 (11%)	50 (14%)	0.41	6 (7%)	6 (7%)	1.000
RENAL score							
≤6	192 (36%)	80 (46%)	112 (31%)	0.005	32 (40%)	32 (40%)	1.000
7–9	228 (43%)	65 (37%)	163 (46%)		37 (46%)	37 (46%)	
≥10	113 (21%)	30 (17%)	83 (23%)		11 (14%)	11 (14%)	
LOS, d	3 (2–5)	2 (2–5)	3 (3–5)	<0.001	2 (2–3)	3 (3–4)	<0.001
Blood transfusions, n (%)	24 (4%)	6 (3%)	18 (5%)	0.40	2 (2%)	5 (6%)	0.25
Postoperative eGFR, ml/min	73.6 (58.9–87.7)	75.7 (60.9–90.9)	72.7 (58.1–86.7)	0.13	76.1 (62.7–89.5)	72.9 (56.3–84.1)	0.15
Postoperative CKD stage							
1–2	397 (75%)	135 (77%)	262 (73%)	0.61	65 (81%)	54 (68%)	0.12
3A–3B	120 (22%)	35 (20%)	85 (24%)		13 (17%)	24 (30%)	
4–5	16 (3%)	5 (3%)	11 (3%)		2 (2%)	2 (2%)	
Trifecta, n (%)	458 (86%)	163 (93%)	295 (83%)	<0.001	77 (96%)	67 (84%)	0.008
pSM, n (%)	8 (1.5%)	3 (1.7%)	5 (1.4%)	0.78	1 (1%)	1 (1%)	0.99
CD ≧ 3 complications, n (%)	21 (4%)	3 (2%)	18 (5%)	0.06	1 (1%)	5 (6%)	0.09
sRFD, n (%)	54 (10%)	10 (6%)	44 (12%)	0.02	2 (2%)	9 (11%)	0.03

SL = sutureless, RR = renorrhaphy, PSM = propensity score-matched analysis, ASA = American Society of Anesthesiologists score, eGFR = estimated glomerular filtration rate, LOS = length of stay, pSM = positive surgical margins, CD = Clavien–Dindo grade, and sRFD = significant renal function deterioration.

Median follow-up time was 17 months (IQR: 8–30): 27 months (IQR: 14–36) in the RR cohort and 9 months (IQR: 6–14) in the SL group.

The PSM analysis generated two cohorts of 80 patients each, homogeneous for age, gender, ASA score, baseline eGFR, tumor size, and RENAL score (all p > 0.12). Patients receiving SL had shorter hospital stays (2 days vs. 3 days; p < 0.001) and increased likelihoods of achieving trifecta (96% vs. 84%; p = 0.008) (Table 1). SMFS probabilities were comparable at KM analysis (log-rank = 0.183) (Figure 1). Multivariable logistic regression analysis identified age (OR: 0.97; 95%CI: 0.95–0.99; p = 0.01), a RENAL score ≧ 10 (OR: 0.29; 95%CI: 0.15–0.57; p < 0.001), and renorrhaphy (OR: 0.34; 95%CI: 0.17–0.67; p = 0.002) as independent predictors of trifecta nonachievement (Table 2). Age at surgery (OR: 1.07; 95%CI: 1.04–1.11; p < 0.001), a RENAL score ≧ 10 (OR: 4.96; 95%CI: 2.23–11.06; p < 0.001), and RR (OR: 2.35; 95%CI: 1.12–4.94; p = 0.02) independently predicted sRFD (Supplementary Materials Table S2). At Cox analyses, age (HR: 1.03; 95%CI: 1.003–1.07; p = 0.03) and baseline eGFR (HR: 0.99; 95%CI: 0.97–0.99; p = 0.05) independently predicted sCKDsm (Table 2).

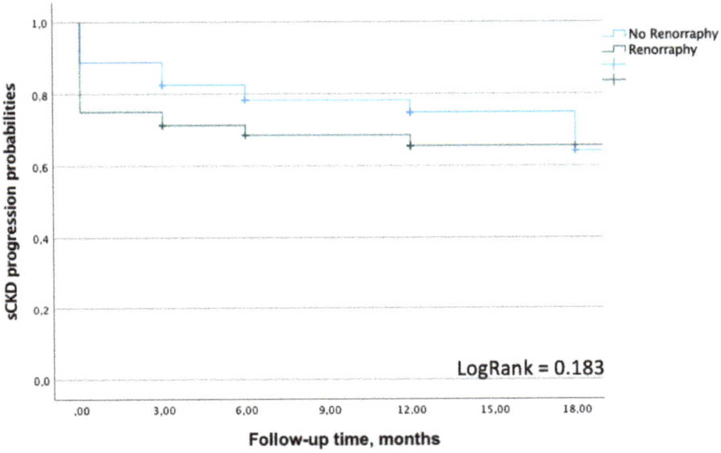

sCKD stage migration-free survival	3 mo	6 mo	12 mo
No Renorraphy			
- Probabilities ± SE	89±3	82±4	75±5
- Number at risk (events)	71 (10)	59 (15)	45 (18)
Renorraphy			
- Probabilities ± SE	75±5	68±5	65±5
- Number at risk (events)	60 (21)	52 (24)	46 (26)

Figure 1. Impact of renorrhaphy on significant CKD stage migration-free survival (SMFS) probabilities after ocRPN.

Table 2. Uni-/multivariable logistic regression analyses to identify predictors of trifecta nonachievement and Cox analyses to identify predictors of significant CKD stage migration.

	Univariable Logistic Regression Analysis to Identify Predictors of Trifecta Achievement				Multivariable Logistic Regression Analysis to Identify Predictors of Trifecta Achievement				Univariable Cox Analysis to Identify Predictors of Significant CDK Stage Migration				Multivariable Cox Analysis to Identify Predictors of Significant CDK Stage Migration			
	OR	95% CI Lower	95% CI Higher	p	OR	95% CI Lower	95% CI Higher	p	HR	95% CI Lower	95% CI Higher	p	HR	95% CI Lower	95% CI Higher	p
Age	**0.98**	**0.96**	**0.99**	**0.03**	**0.97**	**0.95**	**0.99**	**0.01**	**1.04**	**1.01**	**1.07**	**0.003**	**1.03**	**1.003**	**1.07**	**0.03**
Male gender	0.85	0.51	1.41	0.53	-	-	-	-	0.72	0.39	1.34	0.30	-	-	-	-
ASA ≧ 3	0.68	0.39	1.15	0.15	-	-	-	-	1.54	0.79	2.99	0.21	-	-	-	-
Pre-eGFR	1.02	1.02	1.02	<0.001	0.99	0.99	1.01	0.92	**0.98**	**0.97**	**0.99**	**0.006**	**0.99**	**0.97**	**0.99**	**0.05**
RENAL score				**<0.001**				**<0.001**				**0.65**				
≤6	**ref**	-	-		**ref**	-	-		ref	-	-		-	-	-	-
7–9	**0.68**	**0.37**	**1.26**	**0.22**	**0.67**	**0.35**	**1.27**	**0.22**	0.82	0.40	1.68	0.63				
≥10	**0.29**	**0.15**	**0.56**	**<0.001**	**0.29**	**0.15**	**0.57**	**<0.001**	0.40	0.53	2.66	0.39				
Renorrhaphy	**0.31**	**0.16**	**0.60**	**<0.001**	**0.34**	**0.17**	**0.67**	**0.002**	0.87	0.43	1.75	0.69	-	-	-	-

ASA = American Society of Anesthesiologists score. Pre-eGFR = preoperative estimated glomerular filtration rate.

4. Discussion

An average 20% decline in function after NSS is observed in the treated kidney right after partial nephrectomy. Such deterioration is mainly due to a resected healthy parenchymal margin, ischemia/reperfusion damage at the time of hilar clamping, and "reconstructive injury" caused by RR [19]. The first two variables have been extensively investigated, as these were considered the only modifiable factors. A recent multicenter prospective study on 507 NSSs provided evidence that both the resection technique (pure enucleation vs. enucleoresection) and warm ischemia time are independent predictors of postoperative acute kidney injury [20]. As "every minute counts when the renal hilum is clamped during partial nephrectomy" [3], different approaches to minimize hypoperfusion were proposed, such as preoperative superselective transarterial embolization [21], parenchymal [22] or superselective [23] clamping, early unclamping [24], zero ischemia [25], and a purely off-clamp approach [26]. The benefits of these techniques are particularly evident in selected clinical settings, such as patients who are candidates for imperative NSS [27], while for those with a normal eGFR at baseline, their advantage remains controversial.

As said above, the reconstructive injury caused by RR has been considered unavoidable for decades. This, however, is hypothesized to be responsible for 2/3 of the postoperative functional loss [7]. An interesting in vivo study showed that the depth of the necrosis of the renal parenchyma caused by RR ranges between 7 and 15 mm in pigs [8]. Hidas et al. provided evidence that omitting cortical stitching during open partial nephrectomy with cold ischemia provides an advantage in terms of function loss according to postoperative nuclear scans (−11.5% vs. −20.4%; $p = 0.02$) [28]. Similarly, Bahler and colleagues observed a significant volume preservation benefit (−3.8% vs. −15.6%; $p < 0.001$) in patients receiving SL on-clamp RAPN ($n = 38$) compared to those who received RR ($n = 118$); parenchymal suture continued to be an independent predictor of kidney damage according to multivariate analysis ($p < 0.001$) and after PSM analysis ($p = 0.004$) [29].

Since renorrhaphy affects the postoperative glomerular filtration rate and may even cause severe complications, such as pseudoaneurysms and arteriovenous fistulas [9,30], we hypothesized that achieving hemostasis through an SL approach could result in improved functional and surgical outcomes. Actually, electrocauterization has been already successfully employed for the same purposes during liver [31], lung [32], and pancreatic [33] surgeries. In fact, modern electrical scalpels are capable of delivering the proper amount of energy to the tissues so that Joule heat is produced locally, proteins coagulate at a temperature of 70–80 °C, and bleeding stops, while collateral carbonization is limited. A recent Japanese in vivo study tested the effects of electrocautery on a porcine renal model; delivering monopolar energy until hemostasis was achieved, and a 4.6 mm denaturation depth was observed, regardless of cauterization time. Interestingly, a lack or excess of saline solution dripping on the surgical field resulted in an average 2 mm penetration depth and insufficient bleeding control [34]. In 2014, Ota et al. published the first report on the use of coagulation during 39 laparoscopic partial nephrectomies (LPNs) (two-thirds were on-clamp NSSs); all operations were uneventful, and none required blood transfusions or conversion to nephrectomy. Eleven cases (28%), though, necessitated intraoperative repair of the collecting system. No significant decrease in renal function was observed within the study period [35]. Similar results were reported by Hongo et al. in a series of 32 off-clamp LPNs [36]. In 2019, Tohi and colleagues compared outcomes of SL on-clamp RAPN for cT1a ($n = 66$) and cT1b renal masses ($n = 34$); as expected, operation (154 vs. 184 min; $p < 0.001$) and ischemia times (14 vs. 21 min; $p < 0.001$) appeared significantly longer in the latter cohort, while the rate of positive surgical margin was comparable in the two groups (4.5% vs. 11.7%; $p = 0.22$). Of note, three major complications were observed, and all occurred in the cohort with larger tumors [37]. Two other small retrospective controlled studies showed a benefit in renal function and volume preservation when omitting cortical renorrhaphy during minimally invasive NSS [30,38].

In the present paper, we report outcomes of a continuous series of patients who underwent ocRAPN at our center. From January 2020, all those presenting with a cT1-

2N0M0 renal mass that was suitable for ocRAPN were treated with an SL intent; 10/180 cases (5%) required RR because of an intraoperative suspicion of iatrogenic renal calyx injury ($n = 8$) or uncontrollable bleeding ($n = 2$). The latter presented with large (median tumor size: 4.7 cm; IQR: 3–6) and complex (60% had a RENAL score of 7–9; 40% had a RENAL score $\geq$ 10) neoplasms (Supplementary Materials). Most of the patients in the SL group harbored small (3 cm; IQR: 2.5–5), uncomplex renal tumors (83% had a RENAL score <10), and less than one out of five presented with an ASA score $\geqq$ 3. When compared to patients from the RR cohort (whose baseline characteristics were slightly, though not significantly, worse), the former reported a higher trifecta rate (93% vs. 83%; $p < 0.001$), and this difference was confirmed after PSM analysis (96% vs. 84%; $p = 0.008$) (Table 1). Interestingly, the multivariable logistic regression analysis confirmed that RR significantly reduces the probabilities of achieving trifecta (OR: 0.34; 95%CI: 0.17–0.67; $p = 0.002$), together with age (OR: 0.97; 95%CI: 0.95–0.99; $p = 0.01$) and a RENAL score $\geqq$ 10 (OR: 0.29; 95%CI: 0.15–0.57; $p < 0.001$) (Table 2). Of note, the rate of sRFD was significantly reduced in the SL cohort (6% vs. 12%; $p = 0.02$) (Table 1), but this advantage, in terms of kidney function preservation, was only observed at hospital discharge and did not translate to a reduced risk of sCKD stage migration at a 12-month follow-up (Table 2, Figure 1). In fact, only age (HR: 1.03; 95%CI: 1.003–1.07; $p = 0.03$) and preoperative eGFR (HR: 0.99; 95%CI: 0.97–0.99; $p = 0.05$) independently predicted a significant worsening of renal function at Cox analysis.

Additionally, the rates of CD grade $\geqq$3 complications (2% vs. 5%; $p = 0.12$), transfusions (3% vs. 4%; $p = 0.62$), and urinary fistulas (2% vs. 1%; $p = 0.18$) were comparable in the two groups, and were in line with other published series concerning ocRAPN [17]. These findings are of particular interest, considering that there are reports of urinomas due to coagulation in LPN [36,38], and it was consequently suggested to exclude from an SL approach all the patients presenting with a renal mass whose distance to the collecting system was < 5 mm; cautery, in fact, could slow the healing of heat-damaged tissues and make it harder to suture iatrogenic lesions of renal calyces [39].

It is worth highlighting that RR was an independent predictor of the risk of sRFD (OR: 2.35; 95%CI: 1.12–4.94; $p = 0.02$), together with age at surgery (OR: 1.07; 95%CI: 1.04–1.11; $p < 0.001$) and a RENAL score $\geqq$ 10 (OR: 4.96; 95%CI: 2.23–11.06; $p < 0.001$). These results are in line with the available literature; in fact, it was hypothesized that the reconstructive injury caused by stitching the parenchymal breach may contribute to the postoperative functional loss [7]. Moreover, it is well-known that GFR decreases with age and that older patients have a reduced capability to cope with ischemic kidney damage [13]. Furthermore, there is strong evidence that highly complex tumors are associated with an increased contact surface area, which in turn requires more energy (in the case of an SL approach) or stitches (when RR is performed) to achieve hemostasis [11], thus increasing the risk of damaging the remaining healthy parenchyma. Surprisingly, our logistic regression analyses failed to prove any association between gender and the response to renal injury; in fact, there is evidence that women may be more protected against temporarily impaired renal circulation [40,41].

To the best of our knowledge, the series of RAPNs herein reported is the first ever published with an SL purely off-clamp approach. This study, however, suffers from the limitations inherent to its retrospective design; because of this, it should be considered as a hypothesis-generating study, and results from a randomized controlled trial are awaited in order to assess the possible advantages of any of the two techniques. Moreover, most of the patients in the SL group harbored small (3 cm; IQR: 2.5–5), uncomplex renal tumors (83% had a RENAL score <10), and less than one out of five presented with an ASA score $\geqq$ 3; this significantly limits the generalizability of our findings. Furthermore, to evaluate the potential benefits of this procedure on long-term outcomes, a longer follow-up is required. Another limitation of the present study is that the two groups were not homogeneous in terms of the surgeon's experience with the two techniques. In fact, in 2017, G.S. had already completed his learning curve with the conventional RR-ocRAPN; on the contrary, the SL approach was only introduced in 2020, and the very first cases performed with this novel technique were included in the present analysis. Another possible bias is the lack of strict criteria to select patients for the SL approach; at our center, all the patients harboring a cT1-2N0M0 renal mass suitable for NSS are offered an ocRAPN, and the indication for RR is currently decided during surgery, in case of profuse incoercible bleeding or iatrogenic injury of the collecting system. Consequently, our control group also included patients who were not theoretically eligible for both approaches but strictly necessitated the RR.

5. Conclusions

The patients in our study who, after 2020, received sutureless RAPN without hilum dissection and clamping, showed a good safety profile, low complications, and reduced incidence of perioperative and short-term renal function decrease. In our hands, and in the cases shown in this study, the sutureless technique, associated with monopolar coagulation of the resected bed, was associated with a statistically significant increase in trifecta achievement, as compared to standard renorrhaphy cases. Although our results are encouraging and stimulate further investigation, a larger study group, patients' randomization, renal scan-based assessment of renal function, and longer follow-up are required before drawing definite conclusions on the potential long-term benefit of our proposed technique in kidney cancer surgery.

Supplementary Materials: The following supporting information can be downloaded at: https://www.mdpi.com/article/10.3390/cancers15030698/s1.

Author Contributions: Conceptualization, A.B. and G.S.; data curation, L.M., U.A., A.M.B., M.C. (Manuela Costantini), M.C.F., R.M., G.T. (Giulia Torregiani), M.C. (Marco Covotta), and G.T. (Gabriele Tuderti); formal analysis, A.B. and G.S.; supervision, S.G. and G.S.; visualization, L.M. and G.S.; writing—original draft, A.B.; writing—review and editing, A.B. and G.S. All authors have read and agreed to the published version of the manuscript.

Funding: This research received no external funding.

Institutional Review Board Statement: This study was conducted according to the guidelines of the Declaration of Helsinki and approved by the Institutional Review Board of IRE (protocol code M.BBIRE.02 and date of approval 26 March 2017).

Informed Consent Statement: Informed consent was obtained from all subjects involved in this study.

Data Availability Statement: Data supporting reported results are deposited at https://gbox.garr.it/garrbox/index.php/s/w4XVqbXO7CgdwH4 accessed on 18 January 2023.

Conflicts of Interest: The authors declare no conflict of interest.

References

1. Simone, G.; De Nunzio, C.; Ferriero, M.; Cindolo, L.; Brookman-May, S.; Papalia, R.; Sperduti, I.; Collura, D.; Leonardo, C.; Anceschi, U.; et al. Trends in the Use of Pa0rtial Nephrectomy for CT1 Renal Tumors: Analysis of a 10-Yr European Multicenter Dataset. *Eur. J. Surg. Oncol.* **2016**, *42*, 1729–1735. [CrossRef] [PubMed]
2. Lane, B.R.; Demirjian, S.; Derweesh, I.H.; Takagi, T.; Zhang, Z.; Velet, L.; Ercole, C.E.; Fergany, A.F.; Campbell, S.C. Survival and Functional Stability in Chronic Kidney Disease Due to Surgical Removal of Nephrons: Importance of the New Baseline Glomerular Filtration Rate. *Eur. Urol.* **2015**, *68*, 996–1003. [CrossRef] [PubMed]
3. Thompson, R.H.; Lane, B.R.; Lohse, C.M.; Leibovich, B.C.; Fergany, A.; Frank, I.; Gill, I.S.; Blute, M.L.; Campbell, S.C. Every Minute Counts When the Renal Hilum Is Clamped during Partial Nephrectomy. *Eur. Urol.* **2010**, *58*, 340–345. [CrossRef] [PubMed]
4. Desai, M.M.; De Castro Abreu, A.L.; Leslie, S.; Cai, J.; Huang, E.Y.H.; Lewandowski, P.M.; Lee, D.; Dharmaraja, A.; Berger, A.K.; Goh, A.; et al. Robotic Partial Nephrectomy with Superselective versus Main Artery Clamping: A Retrospective Comparison. *Eur. Urol.* **2014**, *66*, 713–719. [CrossRef] [PubMed]
5. Peyronnet, B.; Baumert, H.; Mathieu, R.; Masson-Lecomte, A.; Grassano, Y.; Roumiguié, M.; Massoud, W.; Abd El Fattah, V.; Bruyère, F.; Droupy, S.; et al. Early Unclamping Technique during Robot-Assisted Laparoscopic Partial Nephrectomy Can Minimise Warm Ischaemia without Increasing Morbidity. *BJU Int.* **2014**, *114*, 741–747. [CrossRef]

6. Bertolo, R.; Simone, G.; Garisto, J.; Nakhoul, G.; Armanyous, S.; Agudelo, J.; Costantini, M.; Tuderti, G.; Gallucci, M.; Kaouk, J. Off-Clamp vs on-Clamp Robotic Partial Nephrectomy: Perioperative, Functional and Oncological Outcomes from a Propensity-Score Matching between Two High-Volume Centers. *Eur. J. Surg. Oncol.* **2019**, *45*, 1232–1237. [CrossRef]
7. Bahler, C.D.; Sundaram, C.P. Effect of Renal Reconstruction on Renal Function after Partial Nephrectomy. *J. Endourol.* **2016**, *30*, S37–S41. [CrossRef]
8. Rouach, Y.; Delongchamps, N.B.; Patey, N.; Fontaine, E.; Timsit, M.O.; Thiounn, N.; Méjean, A. Suture or Hemostatic Agent during Laparoscopic Partial Nephrectomy? A Randomized Study Using a Hypertensive Porcine Model. *Urology* **2009**, *73*, 172–177. [CrossRef]
9. Singh, D.; Gill, I.S. Renal Artery Pseudoaneurysm Following Laparoscopic Partial Nephrectomy. *J. Urol.* **2005**, *174*, 2256–2259. [CrossRef]
10. Simone, G.; Papalia, R.; Guaglianone, S.; Gallucci, M. "Zero Ischaemia", Sutureless Laparoscopic Partial Nephrectomy for Renal Tumours with a Low Nephrometry Score. *BJU Int.* **2012**, *110*, 124–130. [CrossRef]
11. Kutikov, A.; Smaldone, M.C.; Egleston, B.L.; Manley, B.J.; Canter, D.J.; Simhan, J.; Boorjian, S.A.; Viterbo, R.; Chen, D.Y.T.; Greenberg, R.E.; et al. Anatomic Features of Enhancing Renal Masses Predict Malignant and High-Grade Pathology: A Preoperative Nomogram Using the RENAL Nephrometry Score. *Eur. Urol.* **2011**, *60*, 241–248. [CrossRef] [PubMed]
12. Inker, L.A.; Schmid, C.H.; Tighiouart, H.; Eckfeldt, J.H.; Feldman, H.I.; Greene, T.; Kusek, J.W.; Manzi, J.; Van Lente, F.; Zhang, Y.L.; et al. Estimating Glomerular Filtration Rate from Serum Creatinine and Cystatin C. *N. Engl. J. Med.* **2012**, *367*, 20–29. [CrossRef] [PubMed]
13. Coresh, J.; Astor, B.C.; Greene, T.; Eknoyan, G.; Levey, A.S. Prevalence of Chronic Kidney Disease and Decreased Kidney Function in the Adult US Population: Third National Health and Nutrition Examination Survey. *Am. J. Kidney Dis. Off. J. Natl. Kidney Found.* **2003**, *41*, 1–12. [CrossRef] [PubMed]
14. Brassetti, A.; Anceschi, U.; Bertolo, R.; Ferriero, M.; Tuderti, G.; Capitanio, U.; Larcher, A.; Garisto, J.; Antonelli, A.; Mottire, A.; et al. Surgical Quality, Cancer Control and Functional Preservation: Introducing a Novel Trifecta for Robot-Assisted Partial Nephrectomy. *Minerva Urol. E Nefrol. Ital. J. Urol. Nephrol.* **2019**, *72*, 82–90. [CrossRef]
15. Levey, A.S.; Inker, L.A.; Matsushita, K.; Greene, T.; Willis, K.; Lewis, E.; De Zeeuw, D.; Cheung, A.K.; Coresh, J. GFR Decline as an End Point for Clinical Trials in CKD: A Scientific Workshop Sponsored by the National Kidney Foundation and the US Food and Drug Administration. *Am. J. Kidney Dis. Off. J. Natl. Kidney Found.* **2014**, *64*, 821–835. [CrossRef]
16. Dindo, D.; Demartines, N.; Clavien, P.-A. Classification of Surgical Complications: A New Proposal with Evaluation in a Cohort of 6336 Patients and Results of a Survey. *Ann. Surg.* **2004**, *240*, 205–213. [CrossRef]
17. Simone, G.; Misuraca, L.; Tuderti, G.; Minisola, F.; Ferriero, M.; Romeo, G.; Costantini, M.; Al-Rawashdah, S.F.; Guaglianone, S.; Gallucci, M. Purely Off-Clamp Robotic Partial Nephrectomy: Preliminary 3-Year Oncological and Functional Outcomes. *Urology* **2018**, *25*, 606–614. [CrossRef]
18. Brassetti, A.; Cacciamani, G.E.; Mari, A.; Garisto, J.D.; Bertolo, R.; Sundaram, C.P.; Derweesh, I.; Bindayi, A.; Dasgupta, P.; Porter, J.; et al. On-Clamp vs. Off-Clamp Robot-Assisted Partial Nephrectomy for CT2 Renal Tumors: Retrospective Propensity-Score-Matched Multicenter Outcome Analysis. *Cancers* **2022**, *14*, 4431. [CrossRef]
19. Mir, M.C.; Ercole, C.; Takagi, T.; Zhang, Z.; Velet, L.; Remer, E.M.; Demirjian, S.; Campbell, S.C. Decline in Renal Function after Partial Nephrectomy: Etiology and Prevention. *J. Urol.* **2015**, *193*, 1889–1898. [CrossRef]
20. Minervini, A.; Campi, R.; Lane, B.R.; De Cobelli, O.; Sanguedolce, F.; Hatzichristodoulou, G.; Antonelli, A.; Noyes, S.; Mari, A.; Rodriguez-Faba, O.; et al. Impact of Resection Technique on Perioperative Outcomes and Surgical Margins after Partial Nephrectomy for Localized Renal Masses: A Prospective Multicenter Study. *J. Urol.* **2020**, *203*, 496–504. [CrossRef]
21. Simone, G.; Papalia, R.; Guaglianone, S.; Carpanese, L.; Gallucci, M. Zero Ischemia Laparoscopic Partial Nephrectomy After Superselective Transarterial Tumor Embolization for Tumors with Moderate Nephrometry Score: Long-Term Results of a Single-Center Experience. *J. Endourol.* **2011**, *25*, 1443–1446. [CrossRef] [PubMed]
22. Simon, J.; Bartsch, G.; Finter, F.; Hautmann, R.; De Petriconi, R. Laparoscopic Partial Nephrectomy with Selective Control of the Renal Parenchyma: Initial Experience with a Novel Laparoscopic Clamp. *BJU Int.* **2009**, *103*, 805–808. [CrossRef] [PubMed]
23. Shao, P.; Qin, C.; Yin, C.; Meng, X.; Ju, X.; Li, J.; Lv, Q.; Zhang, W.; Xu, Z. Laparoscopic Partial Nephrectomy with Segmental Renal Artery Clamping: Technique and Clinical Outcomes. *Eur. Urol.* **2011**, *59*, 849–855. [CrossRef] [PubMed]
24. Nguyen, M.M.; Gill, I.S. Halving Ischemia Time during Laparoscopic Partial Nephrectomy. *J. Urol.* **2008**, *179*, 627–632. [CrossRef] [PubMed]
25. Gill, I.S.; Eisenberg, M.S.; Aron, M.; Berger, A.; Ukimura, O.; Patil, M.B.; Campese, V.; Thangathurai, D.; Desai, M.M. "Zero Ischemia" Partial Nephrectomy: Novel Laparoscopic and Robotic Technique. *Eur. Urol.* **2011**, *59*, 128–134. [CrossRef] [PubMed]
26. Simone, G.; Gill, I.S.; Mottrie, A.; Kutikov, A.; Patard, J.J.; Alcaraz, A.; Rogers, C.G. Indications, Techniques, Outcomes, and Limitations for Minimally Ischemic and off-Clamp Partial Nephrectomy: A Systematic Review of the Literature. *Eur. Urol.* **2015**, *68*, 632–640. [CrossRef] [PubMed]
27. Anceschi, U.; Brassetti, A.; Bertolo, R.; Tuderti, G.; Ferriero, M.C.; Mastroianni, R.; Flammia, R.S.; Costantini, M.; Kaouk, J.; Leonardo, C.; et al. On-Clamp versus Purely off-Clamp Robot-Assisted Partial Nephrectomy in Solitary Kidneys: Comparison of Perioperative Outcomes and Chronic Kidney Disease Progression at Two High- Volume Centers. *Minerva Urol. E Nefrol. Ital. J. Urol. Nephrol.* **2020**, *73*, 739–745. [CrossRef]

28. Hidas, G.; Lupinsky, L.; Kastin, A.; Moskovitz, B.; Groshar, D.; Nativ, O. Functional Significance of Using Tissue Adhesive Substance in Nephron-Sparing Surgery: Assessment by Quantitative SPECT of 99m Tc-Dimercaptosuccinic Acid Scintigraphy. *Eur. Urol.* **2007**, *52*, 785–790. [CrossRef]
29. Bahler, C.D.; Clint Cary, K.; Garg, S.; DeRoo, E.M.; Tabib, C.H.; Kansal, J.K.; Francesca Monn, M.; Flack, C.K.; Masterson, T.A.; Kumar Sandrasegaran, M.; et al. Differentiating Reconstructive Techniques in Partial Nephrectomy: A Propensity Score Analysis. *Can. J. Urol.* **2015**, *22*, 7788–7796.
30. Tohi, Y.; Murata, S.; Makita, N.; Suzuki, I.; Kubota, M.; Sugino, Y.; Inoue, K.; Ueda, H.; Kawakita, M. Absence of Asymptomatic Unruptured Renal Artery Pseudoaneurysm on Contrast-Enhanced Computed Tomography after Robot-Assisted Partial Nephrectomy without Parenchymal Renorrhaphy. *Asian J. Urol.* **2020**, *7*, 24–28. [CrossRef]
31. Itoh, S.; Fukuzawa, K.; Shitomi, Y.; Okamoto, M.; Kinoshita, T.; Taketomi, A.; Shirabe, K.; Wakasugi, K.; Maehara, Y. Impact of the VIO System in Hepatic Resection for Patients with Hepatocellular Carcinoma. *Surg. Today* **2012**, *42*, 1176–1182. [CrossRef] [PubMed]
32. Uchiyama, A.; Miyoshi, K.; Nakamura, K. VIO Soft-Coagulation System for Major Pulmonary Resections: Results in 68 Patients with Primary Lung Cancer. *Gen. Thorac. Cardiovasc. Surg.* **2011**, *59*, 175–178. [CrossRef] [PubMed]
33. Nagakawa, Y.; Tsuchida, A.; Saito, H.; Tohyama, Y.; Matsudo, T.; Kawakita, H.; Ikeda, T.; Kasuya, K.; Ozawa, T.; Aoki, T. The VIO Soft-Coagulation System Can Prevent Pancreatic Fistula Following Pancreatectomy. *J. Hepato-Biliary-Pancreat. Surg.* **2008**, *15*, 359–365. [CrossRef] [PubMed]
34. Fujisaki, A.; Takayama, T.; Teratani, T.; Kubo, T.; Kamei, J.; Sugihara, T.; Ando, S.; Morita, T.; Fujimura, T. Histological and Radiological Evaluation of Thermal Denaturation Depth Using Soft Coagulation during Partial Nephrectomy in Living Pigs. *Int. J. Urol. Off. J. Jpn. Urol. Assoc.* **2021**, *28*, 1274–1280. [CrossRef] [PubMed]
35. Ota, T.; Komori, H.; Rii, J.; Ochi, A.; Suzuki, K.; Shiga, N.; Nishiyama, H. Soft Coagulation in Partial Nephrectomy without Renorrhaphy: Feasibility of a New Technique and Early Outcomes. *Int. J. Urol.* **2014**, *21*, 244–247. [CrossRef] [PubMed]
36. Hongo, F.; Kawauchi, A.; Ueda, T.; Fujihara-Iwata, A.; Nakamura, T.; Naya, Y.; Kamoi, K.; Okihara, K.; Miki, T.; Fumiya, H.M.D. Laparoscopic Off-Clamp Partial Nephrectomy Using Soft Coagulation. *Int. J. Urol.* **2015**, *22*, 731–734. [CrossRef]
37. Tohi, Y.; Murata, S.; Makita, N.; Suzuki, I.; Kubota, M.; Sugino, Y.; Inoue, K.; Kawakita, M. Comparison of Perioperative Outcomes of Robot-Assisted Partial Nephrectomy without Renorrhaphy: Comparative Outcomes of CT1a versus CT1b Renal Tumors. *Int. J. Urol.* **2019**, *26*, 885–889. [CrossRef]
38. Yoshida, T.; Okinaka, Y.; Tomita, K.; Tsuru, T.; Kageyama, S.; Narita, M.; Kawauchi, A. Off-Clamp Tumor Excision Using Soft Coagulation in Laparoscopic and Robotic Partial Nephrectomy. *Asian J. Endosc. Surg.* **2020**, *13*, 519–525. [CrossRef]
39. Naito, S.; Nakashima, M.; Kimoto, Y.; Nakamura, M.; Kotoh, S.; Tanaka, M.; Kumazawa, J. Application of Microwave Tissue Coagulator in Partial Nephrectomy for Renal Cell Carcinoma. *J. Urol.* **1998**, *159*, 960–962. [CrossRef]
40. Ishiyama, Y.; Kondo, T.; Ishihara, H.; Yoshida, K.; Iizuka, J.; Tanabe, K.; Takagi, T. Association between Ureteral Clamping Time and Acute Kidney Injury during Robot-Assisted Radical Cystectomy. *Curr. Oncol.* **2021**, *28*, 4986–4997. [CrossRef]
41. Mancini, M.; Righetto, M.; Baggio, G. Gender-Related Approach to Kidney Cancer Management: Moving Forward. *Int. J. Mol. Sci.* **2020**, *21*, 3378. [CrossRef] [PubMed]

cancers

MDPI

Article

Last Resort from Nursing Shortage? Comparative Cost Analysis of Open vs. Robot-Assisted Partial Nephrectomies with a Focus on the Costs of Nursing Care

Philip Zeuschner [1,*], Carolin Böttcher [1], Lutz Hager [2], Johannes Linxweiler [1], Michael Stöckle [1] and Stefan Siemer [1]

1 Department of Urology and Pediatric Urology, Saarland University, 66123 Homburg, Saarland, Germany
2 SRH Distance Learning University, Kirchstraße 26, 88499 Riedlingen, Germany
* Correspondence: philip.zeuschner@uks.eu

Simple Summary: As robotic surgery is less invasive and patients recover faster compared to open surgery, the postoperative nursing effort should be lower. However, this potential cost savings mechanism for the otherwise more expensive robotic surgery has not been investigated yet. Therefore, we compared 198 robotic and 61 open partial kidney resections performed within two years at an experienced center. Indeed, the median total nursing time and daily nursing effort were significantly lower after robotic surgery, which resulted in mean savings of EUR 186.48 in nursing costs per robotic surgery. However, this cost savings mechanism alone did not amortize the overall increased costs of the robotic system.

Abstract: Despite perioperative advantages, robot-assisted surgery is associated with high costs. However, the lower morbidity of robotic surgery could lead to a lower nursing workload and cost savings. In this comparative cost analysis of open retroperitoneal versus robot-assisted transperitoneal partial nephrectomies (PN), these possible cost savings, including other cost factors, were quantified. Therefore, patient, tumor characteristics, and surgical results of all PN within two years at a tertiary referral center were retrospectively analyzed. The nursing effort was quantified by the local nursing staff regulation and INPULS® intensive care and performance-recording system. Out of 259 procedures, 76.4% were performed robotically. After propensity score matching, the median total nursing time (2407.8 vs. 1126.8 min, $p < 0.001$) and daily nursing effort (245.7 vs. 222.6 min, $p = 0.025$) were significantly lower after robotic surgery. This resulted in mean savings of EUR 186.48 in nursing costs per robotic case, in addition to savings of EUR 61.76 due to less frequent administrations of erythrocyte concentrates. These savings did not amortize the higher material costs for the robotic system, causing additional expenses of EUR 1311.98 per case. To conclude, the nursing effort after a robotic partial nephrectomy was significantly lower compared to open surgery; however, this previously unnoticed savings mechanism alone could not amortize the overall increased costs.

Keywords: robot-assisted surgery; partial nephrectomy; nursing shortage; cost analysis; health economics

1. Introduction

Healthcare costs have significantly risen worldwide within the last 15 years, especially in high-income countries [1], partly caused by the increased use of robot-assisted surgical systems [2]. Since their approval in 2000, da Vinci® surgical systems (Intuitive Surgical Inc., Sunnyvale, CA, USA) have spread rapidly worldwide, especially in urologic departments, so that potentially all urologic procedures can be performed with robotic assistance in specialized centers today. For instance, more than 50% of all partial nephrectomies (PN) in the United States were performed with robotic assistance in 2014 [3], and the number of robotic PNs in German hospitals has nearly doubled from 1820 in 2015 to 2989 in 2019 [4].

However, the higher acquisition and running costs compared to open surgery are often not fully reimbursed, depending on the respective healthcare system [5]. The local German Diagnosis Related Groups (DRG) system, for instance, does not cover the higher expenses for the robotic system, which is why various hospital groups did initially not provide robotic surgical systems at all. Nonetheless, a profitable use appears to be possible [6,7]. Some studies even indicate cost savings in high-volume centers compared to open surgery [5,8–10]. Of great importance, lower morbidity, with at least equivalent oncologic outcomes compared with the open approach, has been proven for almost all robot-assisted interventions [11–16].

Beyond the increasing economic constraints, healthcare systems worldwide have recently been subject to further burdens due to the SARS-CoV-2 pandemic which intensified many pre-existing problems. In Germany, there was an increased discourse in the general public about the working conditions of the nursing staff under the catchphrase of a "nursing emergency". Correspondingly, the neologism "Pflexit", the departure of nurses from their professions, was voted third place as the "Word of the Year" in 2021 in Germany [17]. The German legislation has been trying to limit this shortage of nursing staff for some time and the "nursing staff strengthening act" has substantially changed the nursing staff cost reimbursement by outsourcing the nursing staff costs from the G-DRG system in the aG-DRG catalog (a for German word for "excluded").

However, against the background of a nursing shortage on the one hand and increasing economic constraints on the other hand, robot-assisted surgery might open up new opportunities: as robotic surgery is less invasive compared to open surgery, the postoperative nursing effort should be lower. This potential reduction of the workload for the nursing staff and this possible cost-saving mechanism has not yet been investigated and could (partially) amortize the increased material costs. To investigate this hypothesis, all retroperitoneal open vs. transperitoneal robot-assisted partial nephrectomies performed within two years at a tertiary referral center were analyzed in this retrospective, single-center study. In addition to the costs for nursing care, other cost factors were included in this comparative partial cost analysis.

2. Materials and Methods

All open and robot-assisted partial nephrectomies in adults performed at a tertiary referral center for robotic urologic surgery in 2020 and 2021 were retrospectively analyzed. All robotic surgeries were held using a daVinci® X System (Intuitive Surgical Inc., Sunnyvale, CA, USA) via transperitoneal access, and open partial nephrectomies were performed via retroperitoneal access and a flank incision [13]. Immediately postoperatively, all patients were monitored in the urologic intermediate care unit (IMU). They were transferred to the normal ward as soon as they were cardiopulmonary stable, pain compensated, and adequately mobilized. The patients were discharged at sufficient convalescence.

For each patient, demographic factors (i.e., Charlson Comorbidity Index, CCI) and tumor specifics, such as tumor size or PADUA score depicting the tumor complexity, were obtained [15]. The histopathologic reports and intraoperative characteristics, such as warm ischemia time (WIT) were analyzed. Postoperative complications were classified according to the Clavien Dindo Classification and the number of applied erythrocyte concentrates was collected. The surgical outcome was measured using the Trifecta criteria and MIC score (margin, ischemia, and complications) defining the "success" of a partial nephrectomy (MIC: no positive surgical margins, WIT $\leq$ 20 min, no postoperative major complications; trifecta: no positive surgical margins, WIT $\leq$ 25 min, no postoperative complications) [16,17].

The postoperative nursing care effort was quantified via the German nursing staff regulation in the normal ward and via the intensive care and performance recording system (INPULS®) in the IMU or intensive care unit (ICU) [18]. Both systems were developed to measure the patient-specific nursing effort in different dimensions. For the INPULS system, each patient is assigned to one out of six nursing categories per 24 h with respective nursing minute values defining the actual nursing care effort (Table S1). The INPULS system also enables the accurate recording of the occupancy time of a patient in the IMU or ICU, resulting in exact nursing minute values per patient.

For the partial cost analysis, the costs for nursing care, administration of erythrocyte concentrates, and material and consumption costs, including sterilization to perform an average robot-assisted or open PN within the analyzed period, were calculated. The German aG-DRG "L13B", based on the local base-case value, was applied as revenue. With regard to the nursing effort, the hospital-specific nursing charge value of EUR 163.09 per day was applied based on §15 paragraph 2a of the German hospital remuneration act. For the consumables, all materials prepared for surgery by the surgical staff by the standard were assessed. The sterilization costs were calculated in sterile goods units. The analysis was carried out from a case- and occupancy-related perspective.

The statistical analysis was performed using IBM SPSS Statistics System Version 23 (International Business Corporation, Armonk, New York, NY, USA). Categorical (absolute, relative frequency) and continuous (median, range) variables were differentiated. A 1:1 nearest-neighbor propensity score matching was performed with the Charlson Comorbidity Index and PADUA score as matching variables, and the tolerance rate was set to 0.05. Group comparisons were carried out with Fisher's exact test, chi-square, Mann–Whitney U, sign tests, McNemar, and Wilcoxon tests. All tests were two-sided and $p < 0.05$ was considered significant. This work was approved by the responsible ethics committee (Ethics Committee of the Medical Association Saarland, AZ Bu 67/19) and complies with the Declaration of Helsinki (World Medical Association, 2013).

3. Results

Of 259 included patients, 61 (23.6%) underwent open and 198 (76.4%) robot-assisted partial nephrectomies. They were 67.2% male and had a median age of 65 (open) vs. 63 (robotic) years (Table 1). Both groups were comparable in terms of patient characteristics. Patients undergoing open surgery were more comorbid (Charlson Comorbidity Index 10 vs. 7, $p < 0.001$), had more complex (PADUA 9 vs. 8, $p = 0.002$) and by 0.9 cm significantly larger tumors (4.2 vs. 3.3 cm, $p = 0.004$; Table 1).

Table 1. Comparison of patient and tumor characteristics and the histopathological results of open vs. robot-assisted partial nephrectomies (PN) in the overall analysis.

	Open PN (n = 61)	Robotic PN (n = 198)	*p*-Value
patient characteristics			
age	65 (23; 90)	63 (26; 85)	0.151
gender male	41 (67.2%)	133 (67.2%)	1.000
size [cm]	171.5 (152; 195)	174.5 (150; 195)	0.085
weight [kg]	85 (51; 145)	84 (45; 142)	0.939
body-mass index [kg/m²]	27.2 (20.9; 49.6)	28.0 (17.8; 53.0)	0.413
Charlson comorbidity score (CCI)	10 (2; 19)	7 (1; 20)	<0.001
tumor specifics			
PADUA score	9 (6; 13)	8 (6; 12)	0.002
PADUA low risk (6, 7)	11 (18.0%)	55 (27.8%)	0.135
PADUA mid risk (8, 9)	21 (34.4%)	101 (51.0%)	0.028
PADUA high risk (≥10)	29 (47.5%)	42 (21.2%)	<0.001
tumor size [cm]	4.2 (0.9; 12.0)	3.3 (0.5; 9.0)	0.004
malignancy	44 (72.1%)	148 (74.7%)	0.559
pT			0.240
pT1a	25 (41.0%)	93 (47.0%)	0.463
pT1b	10 (16.4%)	42 (21.2%)	0.468
pT2a	2 (3.3%)	2 (1.0%)	0.468
pT3	7 (11.5%)	10 (5.1%)	0.134
pN1	1 (1.6%)	1 (0.5%)	0.774
pR1	6 (9.8%)	16 (8.1%)	0.747
histological subtype			0.093
clear cell	35 (57.4%)	97 (49.0%)	0.305
chromophobe	3 (4.9%)	14 (7.1%)	0.769
papillary	5 (8.2%)	35 (17.7%)	0.103
other malignant	1 (1.6%)	2 (1.0%)	0.555
angiomyolipoma	2 (3.3%)	7 (3.5%)	1.000
oncocytoma	9 (14.8%)	39 (19.7%)	0.454
cyst	2 (3.3%)	1 (0.5%)	0.139

After propensity-score matching, 54 patients per group were compared again without any remaining inherent group differences (Table S2). In the matched analysis, robot-assisted partial nephrectomies lasted significantly longer (open 137.5 vs. robotic 167 min, $p = 0.005$) with a lower proportion of tumor excisions without ischemia (open 31.5% vs. 5.6%, $p = 0.001$; Table 2). The overall complication rate and severity of complications were significantly lower after robot-assisted partial nephrectomy (Table 2). The success rates of Trifecta and MIC were achieved significantly more often after robot-assisted surgery (Trifecta: open 38.9% vs. 75.9%, $p < 0.001$).

Table 2. Comparison of the perioperative outcomes of open vs. robot-assisted partial nephrectomies (PN) after propensity score matching.

	Open PN (n = 54)	Robotic PN (n = 54)	*p*-Value
intraoperative results			
operating time [min]	137.5 (63.5; 286)	167 (77; 342)	0.005
blood loss [mL]	300 (50; 2200)	250 (40; 1500)	0.777
off-clamp excisions	17 (31.5%)	3 (5.6%)	0.001
WIT [min]	15 (5; 30)	13.5 (7; 46)	0.934
conversions			
to open surgery	-	-	
to nephrectomy	3 (5.6%)	0	0.250
postoperative results			
complications	28 (51.9%)	9 (16.7%)	<0.001
Clavien Dindo grade 1	2 (3.7%)	1 (1.9%)	1.000
grade 2	7 (13.0%)	3 (5.6%)	0.344
grade 3a	5 (9.3%)	3 (5.6%)	0.727
grade 3b	11 (20.4%)	1 (1.9%)	0.006
grade 4a	3 (5.6%)	1 (1.9%)	0.625
grade 5	-	-	1.000
erythrocyte concentrate yes	10 (18.5%)	4 (7.4%)	0.146
intraoperative number	0 (0; 1)	0 (0; 2)	0.414
postoperative number	0 (0; 11)	0 (0; 7)	0.082
total number	0 (0; 11)	0 (0; 7)	0.160
Trifecta fulfilled	21 (38.9%)	41 (75.9%)	<0.001
MIC fulfilled	26 (48.1%)	40 (74.1%)	0.008

During the postoperative course, two (3.7%) patients were transferred to the ICU after open partial nephrectomy in the propensity-score-matched analysis, and none after robotic surgery (Table 3). The median length of stay of all patients undergoing open surgery in ICU was zero (range 0–9) days, with an occupancy time of 136.7 (64.5; 208.9) hours and a median nursing effort of 5339.2 (1937.4; 8861) min. On the IMU, the median length of stay after open partial nephrectomy was three (1; 17) days versus one (0; 6) day after robotic intervention ($p < 0.001$). The respective median nursing time of 1305.6 (213.1; 10931.3) min after open partial nephrectomy was more than twice as long compared to robotic surgery ($p < 0.001$). The median length of stay on the normal ward was six (2; 32) vs. four (2; 11) days and was also significantly longer in terms of the nursing effort with 803.5 (70; 4619) vs. 518 (239; 1631) min after open partial nephrectomy ($p < 0.001$). The total nursing time and mean nursing time per day were significantly longer after open partial nephrectomy (open 245.7 vs. 222.6 min, $p = 0.025$).

Table 3. Comparison of the nursing care effort of open vs. robot-assisted partial nephrectomies (PN) in the propensity-score-matched analysis.

	Open PN (n = 54)	Robotic PN (n = 54)	*p*-Value
length of stay [d]			
ICU	0 (0; 9)	-	<0.001
IMU	3 (1; 17)	1 (0; 6)	<0.001
normal ward	6 (2; 32)	4 (2; 11)	<0.001
total	9 (5; 36)	5 (3; 15)	<0.001
occupancy time [h]			
ICU	136.7 (64.5; 208.93)	-	<0.001
IMU	47.5 (7.8; 397.5)	22.1 (0; 140.8)	<0.001
nursing time [min]			
ICU	5399.2 (1937.4; 8861)	-	<0.001
IMU	1305.6 (213.1; 10,931.3)	605 (0; 3.901.5)	<0.001
normal ward	803.5 (70; 4.619)	518 (239; 1631)	<0.001
total	2407.8 (995.1; 12,599.3)	1126.8 (656; 4626.5)	<0.001
nursing time per day [min]	245.7 (160.3; 659.2)	222.6 (131.2; 513.7)	0.025

With average nursing staff costs for a urological nurse of EUR 0.6061 per minute, the daily nursing costs were EUR 148.92 after open vs. EUR 134.92 after robotic partial nephrectomy (Table 4). Against a revenue of EUR 130.60 nursing costs per day, this resulted in a deficit of EUR 18.32 per day after open surgery and a surplus of EUR 21.6 after robotic surgery. As a result of the shorter length of stay after robotic surgery, there was an excess revenue of EUR 186.48 per robotic partial nephrectomy in nursing costs.

Table 4. Comparison of the revenue for nursing care of open vs. robot-assisted partial nephrectomies (PN) in the propensity-score-matched analysis.

	Open PN (n = 54)	Robotic PN (n = 54)
nursing care time/day	245.7 min	222.6 min
nursing costs/day [1]	EUR 148.92	EUR 134.92
revenue/day [2]	EUR −18.32	EUR +4.32
total profit [3]	EUR −164.88	EUR +21.6

[1] based on EUR 0.6061 / nursing minute; [2] based on EUR 130.60 nursing revenue / day; [3] based on length of stay open PN 9, robotic PN 5 days.

At a median consumption of 0.70 erythrocyte concentrates after open and 0.28 after robotic partial nephrectomy, average costs per case of EUR 102.04 and EUR 40.28, respectively, were incurred (Table S3). This corresponded to an excess revenue of EUR 61.76 per robotic partial nephrectomy in costs for erythrocyte concentrates. The material costs per procedure were EUR 1264.55 for robotic and EUR 124.85 for open surgery (Table S4), and average sterilization costs were EUR 164.77 and EUR 104.02, respectively. At average maintenance costs of EUR 357.77 per robotic procedure (for a total of ca. 600 utilizations of the robotic system per year), the total costs resulted in EUR 1789.09 per robotic and EUR 228.87 per open partial nephrectomy.

From a case-related perspective, the reduced nursing effort resulted in a cost savings of EUR 186.58 per robotic partial nephrectomy, in addition to a savings of EUR 61.76 due to less frequent administrations of erythrocyte concentrates (Table 5). These cost savings did not amortize the higher material and consumption costs of EUR 1560.22; additional costs of EUR 1311.98 were incurred. In contrast, from an occupancy-related perspective, the shorter length of stay after a robotic partial nephrectomy resulted in higher revenue potential. During the median length of stay of nine days for an open partial nephrectomy, up to 1.8 times the aG-DRG revenue could be generated within the same time by the robotic procedure, since the length of stay after robotic surgery was shorter. This generated a potential occupancy-related additional revenue of EUR 5615.02 by the robotic approach (Figure 1).

Table 5. Overview of the case-related savings potential of robotic partial nephrectomy.

	Potential Cost Savings
nursing-care costs	EUR +186.48
erythrocyte concentrates	EUR +61.76
material and consumption costs	EUR −1560.22
sum	EUR −1311.98

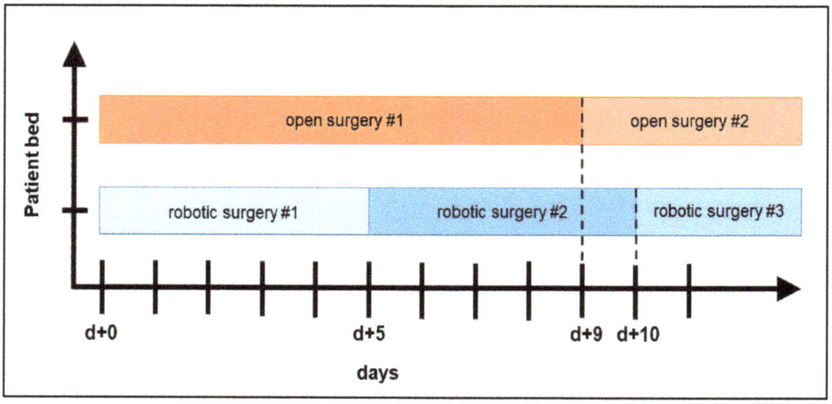

Figure 1. Comparison of robot-assisted vs. open partial nephrectomies from an occupancy-related perspective: in the case of ideal bed occupancy after robotic surgery, its shorter median length of stay enables additional revenue, since more patients can be operated on in the same period.

4. Discussion

Healthcare expenditures worldwide have significantly risen over the past decade, partly due to an increased application of cost-intensive technologies [1,18]. This includes robot-assisted surgery, which is associated with high running and acquisition costs, and has superior perioperative outcomes [19]. Against the background of a significant nursing shortage in some European countries, especially in Germany, the reduced morbidity and a potentially lower nursing workload after a robotic partial nephrectomy might represent a previously unrecognized relief in nursing care and a cost-saving mechanism. To this end, we performed a partial cost analysis with a focus on the nursing care effort of all open vs. robotic partial nephrectomies within the past two years at our department. Ultimately, it was confirmed that the nursing effort was significantly lower after robotic surgery as were the case-related nursing-staff costs. Nevertheless, these savings could not compensate for the additional costs for consumables and sterilization costs associated with the robotic system.

During the analyzed period, a total of 259 partial nephrectomies were held, of which more than 2/3 were performed with robotic assistance. This can be considered a high caseload with an annual number of more than 110 robotic partial nephrectomies in 2021 [20]. The tumor complexity was rather high with nearly 40% high-risk tumors according to PADUA score in the propensity-score-matched analysis [20,21]. In the matched comparison, the operating time was longer after robotic partial nephrectomy. However, there were less frequent and less severe postoperative complications after robotic surgery, the success criteria Trifecta and MIC were achieved more frequently, and the length of stay was shorter. Hence, the results of robotic partial nephrectomy were superior to open surgery [20,22]. Of note, the length of stay after robotic partial nephrectomy underlies multiple factors and can be significantly shorter in other countries. A French working group has recently proven the safety and feasibility of robot-assisted partial nephrectomies in low-risk situations in an outpatient setting [23]. In Germany, this appears rather little attractive, since the revenue of the German diagnosis-related group "L13B" would be significantly shortened as the length of stay would fall below the lower predefined limits.

The hypothesis that the lower morbidity of robotic partial nephrectomy results in a lower nursing workload with potential cost savings could be confirmed in our analysis. The nursing effort was quantified by means of the German nursing staff regulation on the normal wards and the INPULS® categories on the IMU and ICU; it was half as time and labor intensive after robotic partial nephrectomy. Against the background of the differences in length of stay, the mean nursing effort per day was still lower in the robotic group, resulting in savings of EUR 186.46 nursing staff costs per robotic surgery. Of course, it must be questioned whether the minute values adequately reflected the real nursing effort, against the background of other measurement systems for intensive care units. However, the "Therapeutic Intervention Scoring System-28 (TISS-28)" as another common classification system does not adequately reflect the true nursing effort [24,25].

In order to compare these savings with the material costs, a partial cost analysis was performed. To date, two meta-analyses comparing robotic vs. open partial nephrectomies are available. According to Wu et al., the cost difference was not significant, though the costs were slightly higher after robotic surgery [26]. Mir et al. did neither show significant differences, though laparoscopy was found to be the most cost effective [27]. In contrast, Buse et al. estimated that robotic partial nephrectomy was more expensive than open surgery, based on US data reflecting the impact of complications [28]. Shortly thereafter, the same authors concluded in another analysis that the cost of robotic surgery was approximately USD 270 lower [9]. Accordingly, Bahler et al. highlighted in their work at a longitudinal approach that robotic surgery was still USD 1464 more expensive than open surgery in 2009, though already USD 456 cheaper in 2012 [5]; the same was confirmed by Camp et al. for the United Kingdom [29]. In this regard, robotic surgery has become more cost-effective in recent years [10]. A direct comparison of these analyses with our data is difficult since healthcare systems widely differ and the cost factors analyzed here were often ignored in the above-mentioned works. Nevertheless, our estimated values for the sterilization process are similar to those of a French working group [30].

Another highly important cost factor to be analyzed in future investigations is without doubt the costs for the physician staff [31,32]. In 2021, EUR 2000.27 and therewith 28.5% of the total reimbursement for a partial nephrectomy (aG-DRG L13B) was reserved for physician staff costs. Thereof, EUR 780.53 (39%) was addressed for the surgeon during surgery, EUR 525.63 (26.3%) for the anesthetist, EUR 482.47 (24.1%) for medical work on the normal ward, and EUR 79.4 (4%) for physician care on ICU. In order to compare these cost factors between open vs. robot-assisted (vs. potentially laparoscopic) partial nephrectomy in future analyses, the true costs for the surgeon could be deviated from the skin-to-skin time in the operating room, for the anesthetist by the respective anesthesia protocols. However, it will be challenging to estimate the exact time the medical doctors spend with their patients in the normal ward or ICU; in an ideal setting, this could be measured with a stopwatch, which is challenging to implement in the daily routine. As the hourly earnings of medical staff are higher than for nursing, and the postoperative need for medical care is obviously lower after robotic surgery compared to the open intervention, this important cost factor could further reduce the financial gap between open and robotic surgery. However, this hypothesis needs to be confirmed in further work.

Nonetheless, it should be highlighted that our partial cost analysis cannot answer the question whether the robotic partial nephrectomies were *overall* cost covering. Process optimization of robotic partial nephrectomy is certainly not complete against the background of retroperitoneoscopic procedures [33] or potential physician assistants for bedside assistance. With new competitors in the field, such as the HUGO® RAS system (Medtronic, Dublin, Ireland), the costs for robotic systems might continue to decrease in the future [34,35]. In addition, the German aG-DRG reimbursement system is based on cost data from so-called "costing hospitals" which increasingly perform robotic surgery themselves—which is why the reimbursement is expected to continue to increase, as it has significantly risen in recent years for robot-assisted radical prostatectomy [36].

Limitations of this study include the single center setting and a rather short time span, but at a high caseload. Furthermore, the nursing care effort was measured retrospectively. The inherent selection bias was compensated via propensity score matching but reduced the number of cases included in the analysis. Moreover, this analysis only included two specific surgical techniques for partial nephrectomy, namely the retroperitoneal open vs. the transperitoneal robot-assisted access. Partial nephrectomy can also be performed laparoscopically, either at a transperitoneal or at a retroperitoneal approach, but was not included here, since we do not perform laparoscopic partial nephrectomy in our department. Moreover, it is also possible to perform a robot-assisted partial nephrectomy in a retroperitoneoscopic fashion, which has not been established at our institute yet. These different surgical techniques should clearly be investigated in further analyses. Last but not least, only selected cost factors were analyzed—though at high precision; in particular, there are currently no comparable data on postoperative nursing care time and equivalent nursing care costs.

5. Conclusions

It can therefore be concluded that the primary hypothesis of this investigation, namely that the nursing workload was lower after robotic transperitoneal partial nephrectomy compared to retroperitoneal open surgery, could be confirmed. This led to a measurable relief for the nursing staff and clearly represents a previously unknown cost-saving mechanism. However, the respective cost savings, including the less-frequent administration of erythrocyte concentrates, could not amortize the increased material costs of the robotic system—although the question of a cost-covering use of the robotic system was ultimately not answered here. Nevertheless, the increased use of robotic systems in times of a "nursing emergency" in some European countries, such as Germany, could contribute to a lower migration of nursing staff in the future by reducing the daily nursing workload and labor intensity.

Supplementary Materials: The following supporting information can be downloaded at: https://www.mdpi.com/article/10.3390/cancers15082291/s1, Table S1. Overview of the intensive care and performance recording system (Intensivpflege- und Leistungserfassungssystem, INPULS®) and the respective nursing effort-associated categories (modified after (Schöning, 1995)); Table S2. Comparison of patient and tumor characteristics and the histopathological results of open vs. robot-assisted partial nephrectomies (PN) in the propensity score matched analysis; Table S3. Comparison of the average case-related costs for the administration of erythrocyte concentrates after open vs. robot-assisted partial nephrectomy (PN) after propensity score matching; Table S4. Comparison of the average material and consumption costs per partial nephrectomy (PN) after propensity score matching.

Author Contributions: Conceptualization, P.Z. and S.S.; Formal analysis, P.Z. and C.B.; Funding acquisition, P.Z.; Investigation, P.Z. and C.B.; Methodology, P.Z.; Supervision, L.H. and S.S.; Writing—original draft, P.Z.; Writing—review & editing, P.Z., C.B., L.H., J.L., M.S. and S.S. All authors have read and agreed to the published version of the manuscript.

Funding: The research leading to these results received funding from the Intuitive European Research Board under Grant Number 2022-006 UR DE NURS. The Intuitive European Research Board did not interact with the scientific independence of the investigators and did not influence the research. Furthermore, we acknowledge support by the Deutsche Forschungsgemeinschaft (DFG, German Research Foundation) and Saarland University within the "Open Access Publication Funding" program.

Institutional Review Board Statement: This work was approved by the responsible ethics committee (Ethics Committee of the Medical Association of Saarland, AZ Bu 67/19) and complies with the Declaration of Helsinki (World Medical Association, 2013).

Informed Consent Statement: Informed consent was obtained from all subjects involved in the study.

Data Availability Statement: The data that support the findings of this study are available from the corresponding author upon reasonable request.

Conflicts of Interest: Stefan Siemer works as a proctor for Intuitive Surgical. For all other authors, there are no relevant conflicts of interest to declare.

eferences

1. World Health Organisazation. *Global Spending on Health: Weathering the Storm*; World Health Organization: Geneva, Switzerland, 2020; p. 100.
2. Barbash, G.I.; Glied, S.A. New technology and health care costs—The case of robot-assisted surgery. *N. Engl. J. Med.* **2010**, *363*, 701–704. [CrossRef] [PubMed]
3. Flegar, L.; Groeben, C.; Koch, R.; Baunacke, M.; Borkowetz, A.; Kraywinkel, K.; Thomas, C.; Huber, J. Trends in Renal Tumor Surgery in the United States and Germany Between 2006 and 2014: Organ Preservation Rate Is Improving. *Ann. Surg. Oncol.* **2020**, *27*, 1920–1928. [CrossRef]
4. Zeuschner, P.; Siemer, S. Robot-assisted surgery for renal cell carcinoma—Today a standard? *Aktuelle Urol.* **2021**, *52*, 464–473. [CrossRef] [PubMed]
5. Bahler, C.D.; Monn, M.F.; Flack, C.K.; Gramm, A.R.; Gardner, T.A.; Sundaram, C.P. Assessing Cost of Robotic Utilization in Partial Nephrectomy with Increasing Utilization. *J. Endourol.* **2018**, *32*, 710–716. [CrossRef] [PubMed]
6. Rosiello, G.; Palumbo, C.; Deuker, M.; Stolzenbach, L.F.; Martin, T.; Tian, Z.; Larcher, A.; Capitanio, U.; Montorsi, F.; Shariat, S.F.; et al. Partial nephrectomy in frail patients: Benefits of robot-assisted surgery. *Surg. Oncol.* **2021**, *38*, 101588. [CrossRef] [PubMed]
7. Ploussard, G.; Grabia, A.; Barret, E.; Beauval, J.B.; Brureau, L.; Crehange, G.; Dariane, C.; Fiard, G.; Fromont, G.; Gauthe, M.; et al. Annual nationwide analysis of costs and post-operative outcomes after radical prostatectomy according to the surgical approach (open, laparoscopic, and robotic). *World J. Urol.* **2022**, *40*, 419–425. [CrossRef]
8. Probst, K.A.; Ohlmann, C.H.; Saar, M.; Siemer, S.; Stoeckle, M.; Janssen, M. Robot-assisted vs open adrenalectomy: Evaluation of cost-effectiveness and peri-operative outcome. *BJU Int.* **2016**, *118*, 952–957. [CrossRef]
9. Buse, S.; Hach, C.E.; Klumpen, P.; Schmitz, K.; Mager, R.; Mottrie, A.; Haferkamp, A. Cost-effectiveness analysis of robot-assisted vs. open partial nephrectomy. *Int. J. Med. Robot. Comput. Assist. Surg.* **2018**, *14*, e1920. [CrossRef] [PubMed]
10. Baghli, A.; Achit, H.; Audige, V.; Larre, S.; Branchu, B.; Balkau, B.; Eschwege, P.; Hubert, J.; Mazeaud, C. Cost-effectiveness of robotic-assisted surgery vs open surgery in the context of partial nephrectomy for small kidney tumors. *J. Robot. Surg.* **2023**. [CrossRef] [PubMed]
11. Rai, B.P.; Bondad, J.; Vasdev, N.; Adshead, J.; Lane, T.; Ahmed, K.; Khan, M.S.; Dasgupta, P.; Guru, K.; Chlosta, P.L.; et al. Robot-assisted vs open radical cystectomy for bladder cancer in adults. *BJU Int.* **2020**, *125*, 765–779. [CrossRef] [PubMed]
12. Grivas, N.; Kalampokis, N.; Larcher, A.; Tyritzis, S.; Rha, K.H.; Ficarra, V.; Buffi, N.; Ploumidis, A.; Autorino, R.; Porpiglia, F.; et al. Robot-assisted versus open partial nephrectomy: Comparison of outcomes. A systematic review. *Minerva Urol. Nefrol.* **2019**, *71*, 113–120. [CrossRef] [PubMed]
13. Ilic, D.; Evans, S.M.; Allan, C.A.; Jung, J.H.; Murphy, D.; Frydenberg, M. Laparoscopic and robot-assisted vs open radical prostatectomy for the treatment of localized prostate cancer: A Cochrane systematic review. *BJU Int.* **2018**, *121*, 845–853. [CrossRef] [PubMed]
14. Zeuschner, P.; Linxweiler, J.; Mohr, R.; van Heemskerk, S.; Wagenpfeil, G.; Wagenpfeil, S.; Ohlmann, C.; Siemer, S.; Stockle, M.; Saar, M. Robot-assisted versus open radical cystectomy: A cohort study on perioperative outcomes accounting for stage selection bias and surgical experience. *Int. J. Med. Robot.* **2021**, *17*, e2258. [CrossRef] [PubMed]
15. Zeuschner, P.; Greguletz, L.; Meyer, I.; Linxweiler, J.; Janssen, M.; Wagenpfeil, G.; Wagenpfeil, S.; Siemer, S.; Stockle, M.; Saar, M. Open versus robot-assisted partial nephrectomy: A longitudinal comparison of 880 patients over 10 years. *Int. J. Med. Robot.* **2021**, *17*, 1–8. [CrossRef] [PubMed]
16. Kawaguchi, S.; Izumi, K.; Naito, R.; Kadomoto, S.; Iwamoto, H.; Yaegashi, H.; Nohara, T.; Shigehara, K.; Yoshida, K.; Kadono, Y.; et al. Comparison of Clinical Outcomes between Robot-Assisted Partial Nephrectomy and Cryoablation in Elderly Patients with Renal Cancer. *Cancers* **2022**, *14*, 5843. [CrossRef] [PubMed]
17. Tagesschau. "Wellenbrecher" ist das "Wort des Jahres". Available online: https://www.tagesschau.de/inland/wortdesjahres-wellenberecher-101.html#:~:text=2021%201%20Min-,Jury%20der%20%22Gesellschaft%20f%C3%BCr%20deutsche%20Sprache%22%20k%C3%BCrt%20%22Wellenbrecher%22,als%20Wort%20des%20Jahres%202021 (accessed on 6 January 2022).
18. Statistisches Bundesamt. Health expenditures in Germany. Available online: https://www.destatis.de/EN/Themes/Society-Environment/Health/Health-Expenditure/_node.html (accessed on 6 January 2022).
19. Leitlinienprogramm Onkologie (Deutsche Krebsgesellschaft, D.K., AWMF). Konsultationsfassung S3-Leitlinie Diagnostik, Therapie und Nachsorge des Nierenzellkarzinoms, Version 4.0—Februar 2023, AWMF-Registernummer 043/017OL. 2022. Available online: https://www.leitlinienprogramm-onkologie.de/leitlinien/nierenzellkarzinom/ (accessed on 11 April 2023).
20. Peyronnet, B.; Tondut, L.; Bernhard, J.C.; Vaessen, C.; Doumerc, N.; Sebe, P.; Pradere, B.; Guillonneau, B.; Khene, Z.E.; Nouhaud, F.X.; et al. Impact of hospital volume and surgeon volume on robot-assisted partial nephrectomy outcomes: A multicentre study. *BJU Int.* **2018**, *121*, 916–922. [CrossRef]

21. Ficarra, V.; Novara, G.; Secco, S.; Macchi, V.; Porzionato, A.; De Caro, R.; Artibani, W. Preoperative aspects and dimensions use for an anatomical (PADUA) classification of renal tumours in patients who are candidates for nephron-sparing surgery. *Eur. Ur* **2009**, *56*, 786–793. [CrossRef]
22. Cacciamani, G.E.; Medina, L.G.; Gill, T.; Abreu, A.; Sotelo, R.; Artibani, W.; Gill, I.S. Impact of Surgical Factors on Robotic Parti Nephrectomy Outcomes: Comprehensive Systematic Review and Meta-Analysis. *J. Urol.* **2018**, *200*, 258–274. [CrossRef] [PubMe
23. Bernhard, J.C.; Robert, G.; Ricard, S.; Michiels, C.; Capon, G.; Boulenger de Hautecloque, A.; Bensadoun, H.; Gay, J.; Rogier, Tauzin-Fin, P.; et al. Day-case robotic-assisted partial nephrectomy: Feasibility and preliminary results of a prospective evaluatic (UroCCR-25 AMBU-REIN study). *World J. Urol.* **2022**, *40*, 1351–1357. [CrossRef] [PubMed]
24. Glass, F.; Tack, A.K. Personalbedarfsmessung für die Intensivstation. *Pflege Z.* **2021**, *74*, 21–23. [CrossRef] [PubMed]
25. Simon, M. Stellenabbau im Pflegedienst der Krankenhäuser: Mindestanforderungen als Ansatz zur nachhaltigen Sicherung eine ausreichenden Personalbesetzung—Abschlussbericht. 2008. p. 119. Available online: https://www.boeckler.de/pdf_fof/9667 pdf (accessed on 11 April 2023).
26. Wu, Z.; Li, M.; Liu, B.; Cai, C.; Ye, H.; Lv, C.; Yang, Q.; Sheng, J.; Song, S.; Qu, L.; et al. Robotic versus open partial nephrectom A systematic review and meta-analysis. *PLoS ONE* **2014**, *9*, e94878. [CrossRef]
27. Mir, S.A.; Cadeddu, J.A.; Sleeper, J.P.; Lotan, Y. Cost comparison of robotic, laparoscopic, and open partial nephrectomy. *J. Endourc* **2011**, *25*, 447–453. [CrossRef]
28. Buse, S.; Hach, C.E.; Klumpen, P.; Alexandrov, A.; Mager, R.; Mottrie, A.; Haferkamp, A. Cost-effectiveness of robot-assiste partial nephrectomy for the prevention of perioperative complications. *World J. Urol.* **2016**, *34*, 1131–1137. [CrossRef] [PubMed
29. Camp, C.; O'Hara, J.; Hughes, D.; Adshead, J. Short-term Outcomes and Costs Following Partial Nephrectomy in England: A Population-based Study. *Eur. Urol. Focus.* **2018**, *4*, 579–585. [CrossRef] [PubMed]
30. Abd El Fattah, V.; Chevrot, A.; Meusy, A.; Mercier, G.; Wagner, L.; Soustelle, L.; Boukaram, M.; Thuret, R.; Costa, P.; Droupy, S Cost comparison of open and robot-assisted partial nephrectomy in treatment of renal tumor. *Prog. Urol.* **2016**, *26*, 295–303 [CrossRef]
31. Laydner, H.; Isac, W.; Autorino, R.; Kassab, A.; Yakoubi, R.; Hillyer, S.; Khalifeh, A.; Campbell, S.C.; Fergany, A. Simmons, M.; et al. Single institutional cost analysis of 325 robotic, laparoscopic, and open partial nephrectomies. *Urol ogy* **2013**, *81*, 533–538. [CrossRef] [PubMed]
32. Mano, R.; Schulman, A.; Hakimi, A.A.; Sternberg, I.A.; Bernstein, M.; Bochner, B.H.; Coleman, J.A.; Russo, P. Cost comparison o open and robotic partial nephrectomy using a short postoperative pathway. *Urology* **2015**, *85*, 596–603. [CrossRef] [PubMed]
33. Laviana, A.A.; Tan, H.J.; Hu, J.C.; Weizer, A.Z.; Chang, S.S.; Barocas, D.A. Retroperitoneal versus transperitoneal robotic-assisted laparoscopic partial nephrectomy: A matched-pair, bicenter analysis with cost comparison using time-driven activity-based costing. *Curr. Opin. Urol.* **2018**, *28*, 108–114. [CrossRef] [PubMed]
34. Ragavan, N.; Bharathkumar, S.; Chirravur, P.; Sankaran, S.; Mottrie, A. Evaluation of Hugo RAS System in Major Urologic Surgery: Our Initial Experience. *J. Endourol.* **2022**, *36*, 1029–1035. [CrossRef] [PubMed]
35. Liatsikos, E.; Tsaturyan, A.; Kyriazis, I.; Kallidonis, P.; Manolopoulos, D.; Magoutas, A. Market potentials of robotic systems in medical science: Analysis of the Avatera robotic system. *World J. Urol.* **2022**, *40*, 283–289. [CrossRef] [PubMed]
36. Intuitive Surgical. *Krankenhausökonomie & Kostenerstattung—Urologie, Allgemeinchirurgie, Gynäkologie und Thoraxchirurgie 2022*; Intuitive Surgical Inc.: Sunnyvale, CA, USA, 2022.

cancers

MDPI

Article

High BMI and Surgical Time Are Significant Predictors of Lymphocele after Robot-Assisted Radical Prostatectomy

Simon Gloger [1,*], Christian Wagner [2], Sami-Ramzi Leyh-Bannurah [2], Stefan Siemer [3], Madeleine Arndt [3], Jens-Uwe Stolzenburg [4], Toni Franz [4] and Burkhard Ubrig [1]

1 Center for Minimally Invasive and Robotic Urology, Augusta Hospital Bochum, Witten/Herdecke University, Bergstraße 26, 44791 Bochum, Germany
2 Department of Urology, Pediatric Urology and Urologic Oncology, St. Antonius Hospital Gronau, Möllenweg 22, 48599 Gronau, Germany
3 Department of Urology, Saarland University, Kirrberger Str. 100, 66421 Homburg, Germany
4 Department of Urology, University of Leipzig, Liebigstraße 20, 04103 Leipzig, Germany
* Correspondence: s.gloger@augusta-bochum.de; Tel.: +49-234-517-2651

Simple Summary: Robot-assisted prostatectomy is one of the main therapeutic options for localized prostate cancer. Lymphoceles are one of the major causes of complications after robot-assisted radical prostatectomy and pelvic lymph node dissection. Because the data on risk factors for lymphoceles remains unclear and inconclusive, they were investigated in the present study using the data set of the prospective randomized trial ProLy. In this study, high BMI was found to be an independent predictor for the occurrence of lymphoceles and symptomatic lymphoceles. In addition, a longer surgical time proved to be another risk factor for the postoperative occurrence of lymphoceles.

Abstract: Lymphoceles (LC) occur in up to 60% after robot-assisted radical prostatectomy (RARP) and pelvic lymphadenectomy (PLND). In 2–10%, they are symptomatic and may cause complications and require treatment. Data on risk factors for the formation of lymphoceles after RARP and PNLD remain sparse in the urologic literature and are inconclusive to date. The underlying data of this secondary analysis were obtained from the prospective multi-center RCT ProLy. We performed a multivariate analysis to focus on the potential risk factors that may influence lymphocele formation. Patients with LC had a statistically significant higher BMI (27.8 vs. 26.3 kg/m^2, $p < 0.001$; BMI $\geq$ 30 kg/m^2: 31 vs. 17%, $p = 0.002$) and their surgical time was longer (180 vs. 160 min, $p = 0.001$) In multivariate analysis, the study group (control vs. peritoneal flap, $p = 0.003$), BMI (metric, $p = 0.028$), and surgical time (continuous, $p = 0.007$) were independent predictors. Patients with symptomatic lymphocele presented with higher BMI (29 vs. 26.6 kg/m^2, $p = 0.007$; BMI $\geq$ 30 kg/m^2: 39 vs. 20%, $p = 0.023$) and experienced higher intraoperative blood loss (200 vs. 150 mL, $p = 0.032$). In multivariate analysis, BMI $\geq$ 30 kg/m^2 vs. < 30 kg/m^2 was an independent predictor for the formation of a symptomatic lymphocele ($p = 0.02$). High BMI and prolonged surgical time are general risk factors for the development of LC. Patients with a BMI $\geq$ 30 kg/m^2 had a higher risk for symptomatic lymphoceles.

Keywords: robot-assisted radical prostatectomy; lymphocele; symptomatic lymphocele; risk factors; pelvic lymph node dissection; RARP; peritoneal flap

1. Introduction

Bilateral pelvic lymphadenectomy (PLND) is currently recommended as an adjunct to radical robot-assisted prostatovesiculectomy (RARP) for medium- and high-risk prostate carcinomas [1,2]. One of the principal complications of lymphadenectomy is lymphoceles which has been reported in 24–51% of patients after RARP with PLND [3–5].

Whilst most lymphoceles (LC) remain asymptomatic and need no treatment, symptomatic lymphoceles (sLC) require treatment and occur in 2–10% of patients [6]. Typical complications from sLCs include superinfection, leg swelling, deep vein thrombosis, and hydronephrosis [7]. Symptomatic lymphoceles are among the most common reasons for readmission after RARP and PLND [8]. Moreover, most studies have focused on the open retropubic-extraperitoneal surgical approach [9–13].

In recent years, numerous authors have proposed surgical strategies for reducing the incidence of lymphoceles [14–18]. Several groups have examined the effect of bilateral peritoneal flaps (PIFs), which are suture-fixated to the endopelvic fascia, on the formation of LC and sLC [5,6,19–22].

A prospective randomized multicenter double-blind ProLy trial has recently compared patients against those without a PIF and found that PIFs resulted in a significant reduction in the overall incidence of LCs (33% to 22%) and in the incidence of sLCs (8.1% to 3.3%) [7].

The present study aimed to identify potential clinical risk factors for LCs and sLCs through a secondary analysis of the ProLy trial data.

2. Methods

2.1. Study Group

We used the data set from the prospective randomized, double-blind ProLy study [7]. After dropout and loss-to-follow-up, the ProLy study analyzed a total of 475 patients. Data were available for the statistical analysis of this population during the recruitment period from November 2018 to August 2020. The vote of the ethics committee (Aerztekammer Muenster, AZ 2018-451-f-S), as well as the registration in the German Register of Clinical Trials (registration number DRKS00015720), was obtained before the start of the study and covered secondary data analysis.

2.2. Surgical Technique

All RARPs were performed transperitoneal. PLND and the formation of bilateral PIFs were standardized in the study protocols. Randomization was performed intraoperatively after the completion of RARP and PLND. According to the randomization result, the patients had either received PIF or not.

2.3. Data Acquisition and Follow-Up

2.3.1. Preoperative Data Set (Patient-Related Risk Factors)

Patient-related parameters had been prospectively collected at study enrollment and before randomization. The following preoperative data were available for secondary analysis: Body mass index (BMI), prostate volume at admission, initial PSA, American Society of Anesthesiologists (ASA) score, and the Charlson Comorbidity Index (CCI).

2.3.2. Perioperative Data Set (Procedure- and Surgeon-Related Risk Factors)

These included operative time, intraoperative blood loss, intraoperative drain placement, length of hospital stay, the total number of harvested lymph nodes, Gleason grade, ISUP (International Society of Urological Pathology) group, pT stage, pN and R status.

2.3.3. Postoperative Follow-Up

Two follow-up appointments were performed postoperatively at 30 and 90 days. These comprised a thorough history focusing on postoperative complications and abdominal and pelvic ultrasonography with a focus on pelvic lymphocele. Follow-up was performed not by the surgical team but by other physicians trained in ultrasound examinations. The study protocol included daily subcutaneous injections of low-molecular-weight heparin for 4 weeks postoperatively.

2.4. Statistical Analysis

The ProLy data set was analyzed for risk factors contributing to the formation of LC and sLCs. Corresponding analyses were performed for the entire sampled population, the peritoneal flap group, and the control group; to describe the metric variables, we determined the count, median, and interquartile range. The Shapiro–Wilk test was used for these variables to check if they were normally distributed. If the normal distribution assumption was not rejected (p-value < 0.1), a comparison was performed using the t-test. If it was rejected, we applied the Mann–Whitney U test. The distribution of categorical data was described in terms of absolute and relative frequencies. We compared the frequency distributions of a categorical variable of independent groups using the χ^2 square test or Fisher's exact test in case of expected cell frequencies of less than five.

Next, we performed univariate and multivariate analyses to determine potential predictors for the formation of lymphocele and of symptomatic lymphocele. A possible center effect with respect to lymphoceles or symptomatic lymphoceles could be excluded before conducting further analysis. The influence of BMI as one possible predictor was calculated in two different models: both continuously and dichotomized according to obesity as defined ($\geq$30 kg/m^2 vs. <30 kg/m^2). Due to only minimal deviations from the study protocol, no analysis with respect to different heparin use was performed. Multivariate analysis was performed as a stepwise regressive elimination of the independent variables. Because of the small number of events in only eight symptomatic lymphoceles in the peritoneal flap group, we skipped performing logistic regression for this subgroup. All tests were conducted two-sided, and the significance level was set at $p < 0.05$. For all data analyses, Dr. Silke Lange (University of Witten/Herdecke, Germany), a certified biostatistician, SAS® 9.4 statistical software, was used (SAS Institute, Cary, NC, USA).

3. Results

All 475 records from the ProLy study were eligible for analysis. A total of 239 patients had received the peritoneal flap, while 236 patients formed a control group.

3.1. Incidence of Lymphoceles (LCs)

Table 1 shows the frequency distribution of the above-described pre- and perioperative potential risk factors, broken down by patients with and without LC formation: patients with LC presented a statistically significantly higher BMI (27.8 vs. 26.3 kg/m^2, $p < 0.001$). They were more frequently clinically obese with a BMI of more than 30 kg/m^2 (31 vs. 17%, $p = 0.002$). Patients with LC had a significantly longer surgical time of approximately 20 min ($p = 0.001$) and a longer hospital stay (0.3 days; $p = 0.02$).

Table 1. Frequency distribution of the potential risk factors for the occurrence of a lymphocele.

Potential Risk Factor	Patients w/o Lymphocele (n = 338)	Patients with Lymphocele (n = 129)	p
Preoperative variables			
Age (Years, IQR)	66 (60–70)	65 (60–70)	0.8 [a]
BMI (kg/m^2, IQR)	26.3 (24.4–28.7)	27.8 (25.8–30.4)	<0.001 [a]
BMI $\geq$ 30 kg/m^2 (n, %)	58 (17)	39 (30)	0.002 [b]
Prostate volume (mL, IQR)	40 (30–50)	41 (30–60)	0.08 [a]
PSA (ng/mL, IQR)	7.2 (5.2–11)	7.2 (5.3–10.3)	0.8 [a]
Median CCI (SD)	2.2 (0.5)	2.3 (0.5)	0.4 [a]
ASA Score >1 (n, %)	284 (86)	113 (88)	0.6 [b]
ASA Score 3 (n, %)	42 (13)	18 (14)	0.7 [b]
Intra- and perioperative variables			
Surgery time (minutes, IQR)	160 (140–182)	180 (150–200)	0.001 [a]
Blood loss (mL, IQR)	150 (100–250)	150 (100–250)	0.2 [a]
Inpatient length of stay (days, SD)	7.2 (5.3)	7.5 (4.4)	0.02 [a]
Drainage (n, %)	65 (20)	21 (16)	0.5 [b]

Table 1. *Cont.*

Potential Risk Factor	Patients w/o Lymphocele (n = 338)	Patients with Lymphocele (n = 129)	p
Pathological variables			
Total lymph nodes (n, %)	14 (11–19)	14 (11–18)	0.5 [b]
ISUP-GGG ≥3 (n, %)	132 (40)	60 (47)	0.15 [b]
T-stage >pT2 (n, %)	141 (43)	47 (38)	0.3 [b]
Nodal status pN1 (n, %)	25 (8)	10 (8)	0.9 [b]
R1status (n, %)	35 (11)	11 (9)	0.5 [b]

ASA = American Society of Anesthesiologists, BMI = Body mass index, CCI = Charlson comorbidity index, ISUP-GGG = International Society of Urological Pathology—Gleason grading groups, IQR = interquartile range, PSA = prostate-specific antigen, SD = standard deviation. [a] Mann–Whitney U test; [b] χ^2 square test.

We also separately analyzed the treatment group (with PIF) and the control group (without PIF). In the PIF group, BMI (27.6 vs. 26.4 kg/m^2, p = 0.03), obesity (31% vs. 16%, p = 0.02) and surgical time (182 vs. 152 min; p = 0.02) were statistically significant, whereas the length of hospital stay was not (7.6 days vs. 7 days, p = 0.15). In the control group, only a higher BMI (28.8 vs. 26.6 kg/m^2, p = 0.03) was statistically and significantly associated with lymphocele formation.

3.2. Multivariate Analysis (LCs)

In the multivariate analysis of the total study sample (Table 2), randomization (PIF vs. control; p = 0.003), BMI (metric; p = 0.03), and surgical time (p = 0.007) turned out to be independent predictors for LC formation. When separately analyzing the PIF group, only longer surgical time was a predictor of LCs (p = 0.02); in the control group, BMI was an independent predictor of LC formation (metric; p = 0.008).

Table 2. Univariate and multivariate analysis of potential risk factors for the occurrence of lymphocele.

	Univariate				Multivariate			
		95% CI				95% CI		
Potential Risk Factor	OR	Lower Bound	Upper Bound	p	OR	Lower Bound	Upper Bound	p
Preoperative variables								
Age (Years, continuous)	0.99	0.97	1.03	0.9				
BMI (metric)	1.1	1.04	1.15	<0.001	1.07	1.01	1.13	0.03
BMI (≥30kg/m^2 vs. <30kg/m^2)	2.12	1.32	3.39	0.002				
Prostate volume (mL, continuous)	1.01	1	1.02	0.049				
PSA (ng/mL, continuous)	0.99	0.98	1.01	0.7				
CCI (≥1 vs. 0)	1.12	0.78	1.63	0.5				
ASA Score (>1 vs. 1)	1.17	0.64	2.15	0.6				
ASA Score (3 vs. <3)	1.12	0.62	2.02	0.7				
Intra- and perioperative variables								
Surgery time (minutes, continuous)	1.01	1.004	1.01	<0.001	1.01	1.002	1.01	0.007
Blood loss (mL, continuous)	1	1	1.002	0.1				
Length of stay (days, continuous)	1.01	0.97	1.05	0.5				
Study group (Control vs. peritoneal flap)	1.75	1.16	2.64	0.008	1.99	1.26	3.15	0.003
Drainage (yes vs. no)	0.82	0.48	1.4	0.5				

Table 2. *Cont.*

Potential Risk Factor	Univariate				Multivariate			
		95% CI				95% CI		
	OR	Lower Bound	Upper Bound	*p*	OR	Lower Bound	Upper Bound	*p*
Pathological variables								
Total lymph nodes (continuous)	0.99	0.96	1.03	0.6				
ISUP-GGG (3–5 vs. 1–2)	1.02	0.85	1.23	0.8				
T-stage (>pT2 vs. pT2)	0.82	0.54	1.25	0.4				
Nodal status (pN1 vs. pN0)	1.06	0.49	2.27	0.9				
R-status (R1 vs. R0)	0.9	0.52	1.58	0.7				

3.3. *Incidence of Symptomatic Lymphoceles (sLCs)*

sLCs occurred in only 3.3% of the PIF and in 8.1% of the control group. Table 3 shows the frequency distribution of clinical parameters correlated with symptomatic lymphoceles (sLCs). In the total study sample, patients with symptomatic lymphocele had statistically and significantly higher BMI values (29 vs. 26.6 kg/m^2, $p = 0.007$) and a higher proportion of obesity (BMI > 30 kg/m^2, 39 vs. 20, $p = 0.02$). Additionally, the documented intraoperative blood loss was found to be higher (200 vs. 150 mL, $p = 0.03$) compared to patients without symptomatic lymphocele. In the subgroup analysis, with respect to sLCs, none of the clinical parameters reached significant levels in the PIF group. In the control group, only the BMI of patients with a symptomatic lymphocele was significantly higher than that of patients without a symptomatic lymphocele (28.8 vs. 26.6 kg/m^2, $p = 0.03$).

Table 3. Description of patients with and without symptomatic lymphocele.

Potential Risk Factor	Pat. w/o Sympt. Lymphocele (n = 448)	Pat. with Sympt. Lymphocele (n = 27)	*p*
Preoperative variables			
Age (years, IQR)	66 (60–70)	66 (63–72)	0.3 [a]
BMI (kg/m^2, IQR)	26.6 (24.5–29.2)	29 (26.2–32)	0.007 [a]
BMI ≥ 30 kg/m^2 (n, %)	88 (20)	10 (39)	0.023 [b]
Prostate volume (mL, IQR)	40 (30–53)	41 (30–55)	0.7 [a]
PSA (ng/mL, IQR)	7.2 (5.3–10.6)	7.3 (4.8–14.4)	0.9 [a]
Median CCI (SD)	2.3 (0.5)	2.3 (0.5)	0.3 [a]
ASA Score >1 (n, %)	381 (86)	22 (85)	0.8 [c]
ASA Score 3 (n, %)	59 (13)	2 (7.7)	0.4 [c]
Intra- and perioperative variables			
Surgery time (min, IQR)	160 (140–190)	151 (150–182)	0.6 [a]
Blood loss (mL, IQR)	150 (100–250)	200 (150–300)	0.032 [a]
Length of stay (days, SD)	7.3 (5.2)	7 (2.3)	0.3 [a]
Drainage (n, %)	81 (18)	5 (19)	>0.9 [c]
Pathological variables			
Total lymph nodes (n, %)	14 (11–18)	13 (11–20)	0.8 [b]
ISUP-GGG ≥ 3 (n, %)	181 (41)	13 (50)	0.4 [b]

Table 3. *Cont.*

Potential Risk Factor	Pat. w/o Sympt. Lymphocele (n = 448)	Pat. with Sympt. Lymphocele (n = 27)	p
T-stage >pT2 (n, %)	181 (41)	10 (44)	0.8 [b]
Nodal status pN1 (n, %)	33 (10)	2 (8)	>0.9 [c]
R1-Status (n, %)	46 (14)	2 (8)	>0.9 [c]

ASA = American Society of Anesthesiologists, BMI = Body mass index, CCI = Charlson comorbidity index, ISUP-GGG = International Society of Urological Pathology—Gleason grading groups, IQR = interquartile range, PSA = prostate-specific antigen, SD = standard deviation. [a] Mann–Whitney U test; [b] χ^2 square test; [c] Fisher's exact test.

3.4. Multivariate Analysis (sLC)

Obesity (BMI $\geq$ 30 kg/m^2) was an independent predictor for the formation of a symptomatic lymphocele in the total study sample (p = 0.02) (Table 4). In the control group, this was applied to blood loss (p = 0.04). Due to the low incidence (n = 8, 3.3%) of sLC in the PIF group, we did not perform a multivariate analysis on this subgroup.

Table 4. Univariate and multivariate analysis of potential risk factors for the occurrence of symptomatic lymphocele.

	Univariate				Multivariate			
		95% CI				95% CI		
Potential Risk Factor	OR	Lower Bound	Upper Bound	p	OR	Lower Bound	Upper Bound	p
Preoperative variables								
Age (years, continuous)	1.02	0.97	1.08	0.4				
BMI (metric)	1.08	0.99	1.18	0.054				
BMI (≥30 kg/m^2 vs. <30 kg/m^2)	2.53	1.11	5.76	0.027	2.86	1.18	6.9	0.02
Prostate volume (mL, continuous)	1.002	0.98	1.02	0.9				
PSA (ng/mL, continuous)	1.01	0.99	1.03	0.3				
CCI (≥1 vs. 0)	1.19	0.61	2.35	0.6				
ASA Score (>1 vs. 1)	0.87	0.29	2.6	0.8				
ASA Score (3 vs. <3)	0.54	0.12	2.34	0.4				
Intra- and perioperative variables								
Surgery time (min, continuous)	1	0.99	1.01	0.7				
Blood loss (mL, continuous)	1	0.99	1.002	0.3				
Length of stay (days, continuous)	0.98	0.88	1.09	0.7				
Study group (control vs. peritoneal flap)	2.53	1.08	5.9	0.032				
Drainage (yes vs. no)	1.03	0.38	2.8	0.9				
Pathological variables								
Total lymph nodes (continuous)	1.01	0.94	1.08	0.9				
ISUP-GGG (3–5 vs. 1–2)	0.98	0.68	1.4	0.9				
T-stage (>pT2 vs. pT2)	1.11	0.48	2.59	0.8				
Nodal status (pN1 vs. pN0)	1.03	0.23	4.53	0.9				
R-Status (R1 vs. R0)	0.65	0.17	2.55	0.5				

ASA = American Society of Anesthesiologists, BMI = Body mass index, CCI = Charlson comorbidity index, ISUP-GGG = International Society of Urological Pathology—Gleason grading groups, CI = confidence interval, OR = odds ratio, PSA = prostate-specific antigen.

4. Discussion

The present study used data from the prospective randomized ProLy study to investigate risk factors for lymphocele formation after RARP and PLND. In the ProLy study collective, the overall incidence of the lymphocele (LC) was 28% among 475 patients during a follow-up period of 90 days, with 5.7% of the patients developing a symptomatic lymphocele (sLC) [7].

The identification of risk factors seems important for identifying and counseling patients prior to surgery. To date, data on risk factors for lymphocele after RARP and PLND remain scarce and inconclusive in the urologic literature. Furthermore, most of this work relates to the open surgical retropubic approach [9,12,13,23,24].

For robot-assisted RARP, Goßler et al. were able to show an increased risk of lymphocele formation in the presence of a high BMI (OR 1.15, CI 1.05–1.27) in obese patients (OR 2.76, CI 1.05–7.3), aggressive tumors (OR 3.25, CI 1.18–8.92) and an extended operative time (OR 1.01, CI 1.01–1.02) [25]. Another study by Sforza et al. presented higher occurrences of sLC in men with higher BMI (30.4 vs. 25.8 kg/m^2) and a history of vascular surgery (23.8% vs. 8.4%), but only a higher BMI was an independent predictor of sLC after performing multivariate analysis [26]. Similar to the ProLy study, the recently published PerFix study revealed lower incidences of sLC for patients receiving a peritoneal flap (11.5 vs. 2.4%). In their study BMI (OR 1.1, CI 1.03–1.26) and intervention (OR 4.6, CI 1.28–16.82) were independent risk factors for sLC on multivariate analysis [20]. Magistro et al. combined retrospective cohorts of the robotic and retropubic approach of radical prostatectomy and described an increased risk of patients with poorly differentiated tumors (Gleason Score $\geq$ 8) or elevated PSA levels ($\geq$10 ng/mL) as well as for patients with extensive lymphadenectomy (lymph node yield $\geq$ 11) [10].

In our patient sample, we found a significantly increased risk for the formation of lymphoceles in patients with an elevated BMI. This risk factor was valid for the overall incidence of lymphoceles (OR 1.07, CI 1.01–1.13, Table 2) as well as for the occurrence of sLC. Obese patients—when using a BMI $\geq$30 kg/m^2—had almost triple the risk (OR = 2.86, CI 1.18–6.9; p = 0.02) of forming a symptomatic lymphocele (Table 4). This result was consistent with the abovementioned, prospective RCT by Goßler et al. who also found an almost three times higher risk for obese patients (BMI $\geq$ 30 kg/m^2) in developing sLC [25]. Student et al. and Sforza et al. confirmed this finding with their multivariate analyses, demonstrating an OR of 1.1 and 1.7, respectively [20,26]. Intraoperative challenging conditions and chronic inflammation in the adipose tissue could provide reasons for the higher risk of postoperative LC and sLC [25–28]. BMI was also found to be an independent predictor of Clavien 3 complications in patients undergoing RARP with extended PLND [29]. Symptomatic lymphoceles as a major cause of high-grade Clavien-Dindo complications may have been a contributing factor. On the other hand, a study by Mundhenk et al. contrasted with these data, showing that patients with a low BMI had an increased risk of developing symptomatic lymphocele [30]. However, besides being a retrospective report, a limitation of their study is that it did not differentiate between open surgical and transperitoneal robotic-assisted access.

In our study, in addition to BMI, we found increased surgical time to be an independent predictor of lymphocele formation (Table 2). On average, this was 20 min longer (180 vs. 160 min) in patients with the formation of LC than those without. This may indicate a more challenging dissection as potentially favoring lymphocele formation. Our findings are also supported by the already aforementioned study by Goßler and coworkers, who documented this risk factor for symptomatic lymphoceles. They observed an average prolongation of surgical time by 15 min (165 vs. 180 min) in their study sample [25]. Intraoperative blood loss could also be indicative of a more difficult dissection. In our study population, we found significantly higher blood loss in patients who had formed symptomatic lymphocele (Table 3).

The aim of the ProLy study was to investigate the effect of a surgically constructed peritoneal flap (PIF) on lymphocele incidence. The study found that patients with PIF formed significantly fewer LCs (22 vs. 33%) and sLCs (3.3 vs. 8.1%) [7]. As to be expected, on multivariate analysis, the study group was found to be an independent risk factor for the occurrence of LC. Compared to the peritoneal flap group, the control group had a nearly doubled risk (OR 1.99, CI 1.26–3.15; $p = 0.003$) of forming a lymphocele (Table 2). However, on risk factor analysis for the development of sLC, the assignment to the different study group revealed an increased risk for the control group on univariate analysis but did not reach a level of significance on multivariate analysis (Table 4). These data were supported by the PerFix study: Student et al. found the study group to be an independent predictor of symptomatic lymphocele formation with an odds ratio of 4.6 [20]. The study by Goßler et al. differed on this point. Here, the peritoneal flap was not an independent predictor for the development of a symptomatic lymphocele [25].

Additional risk factors such as patient age, the length of lymphadenectomy/number of lymph nodes removed, Gleason grade, or positive nodal status were reported inconsistently and have been discussed controversially in the literature [3,4,11,23,29–31]. In our study, we could not confirm these potential risk factors.

Patients with an ASA score of 2/3 were shown to have a higher incidence of Clavien–Dindo complications greater than one [32]. We also looked at this in our study with respect to lymphoceles or symptomatic lymphoceles as a major cause for high-grade Clavien–Dindo complications but could not confirm this either.

5. Limitations

The main limitation of this data analysis was possibly the small number of symptomatic lymphoceles, which occurred in only 27 patients (5.7%) in the underlying ProLy study. Independent predictors of symptomatic lymphocele may not have been identified due to this small number. Moreover, owing to a small number of symptomatic lymphoceles, multivariate subgroup analysis could not be performed on the peritoneal flap group. Large-scale studies with a higher number of patients would certainly be useful in this regard. Furthermore, the median lymph node yield of the ProLy study was relatively low (14 in each group). Comparable studies had slightly higher lymph node yields (14–17 lymph nodes) [22,33–35]. This may have affected the results and conclusions of the study.

6. Conclusions

In this secondary analysis of the ProLy data set, we found two important independent predictors for lymphocele formation and one for symptomatic lymphocele formation. Obese patients with a BMI ≥ 30 kg/m^2 had a higher risk of symptomatic lymphoceles. Increasing BMI was also correlated with a higher risk for the development of LC. In addition, increasing time spent in surgery was associated with higher incidences of lymphoceles. This could be explained by more challenging surgery conditions resulting in more adverse postoperative events. Therefore, in these patient groups, a close follow-up should be performed in the subsequent postoperative stay and ambulatory care to detect possible complications at an early stage.

Author Contributions: Conceptualization, S.G. and B.U.; methodology, S.G., S.-R.L.-B. and S.S.; writing—original draft preparation, S.G. and B.U.; writing—review and editing, S.S., C.W., S.-R.L.-B., M.A., J.-U.S. and T.F.; visualization, S.S.; supervision, B.U. All authors have read and agreed to the published version of the manuscript.

Funding: This research received no external funding.

Institutional Review Board Statement: The study was conducted in accordance with the Declaration of Helsinki, and was approved by the Ethics Committee of the Aerztekammer Muenster, AZ 2018-451-f-S). It was registered in the German Register of Clinical Trials (registration number DRKS00015720).

Informed Consent Statement: Informed consent was obtained from all subjects involved in the study. Written informed consent was obtained from the patient(s) to publish this paper.

Data Availability Statement: The data presented in this study are available on request from the corresponding author.

Conflicts of Interest: Ubrig: Intuitive Surgery, Procept Biorobotics. Siemer: Intuitive Surgery. The other authors declare no conflict of interest.

References

1. Thompson, I.; Thrasher, J.B.; Aus, G.; Burnett, A.L.; Canby-Hagino, E.D.; Cookson, M.S.; D'Amico, A.V.; Dmochowski, R.R.; Eton, D.T.; Forman, J.D.; et al. Guideline for the Management of Clinically Localized Prostate Cancer: 2007 Update. *J. Urol.* **2007**, *177*, 2106–2131. [CrossRef] [PubMed]
2. Mottet, N.; Bellmunt, J.; Bolla, M.; Briers, E.; Cumberbatch, M.G.; de Santis, M.; Fossati, N.; Gross, T.; Henry, A.M.; Joniau, S.; et al. EAU-ESTRO-SIOG Guidelines on Prostate Cancer. Part 1: Screening, Diagnosis, and Local Treatment with Curative Intent. *Eur. Urol.* **2017**, *71*, 618–629. [CrossRef] [PubMed]
3. Orvieto, M.A.; Coelho, R.F.; Chauhan, S.; Palmer, K.J.; Rocco, B.; Patel, V.R. Incidence of Lymphoceles after Robot-Assisted Pelvic Lymph Node Dissection. *BJU Int.* **2011**, *108*, 1185–1190. [CrossRef] [PubMed]
4. Keskin, M.S.; Argun, Ö.B.; Öbek, C.; Tufek, I.; Tuna, M.B.; Mourmouris, P.; Erdoğan, S.; Kural, A.R. The Incidence and Sequela of Lymphocele Formation after Robot-Assisted Extended Pelvic Lymph Node Dissection. *BJU Int.* **2016**, *118*, 127–131. [CrossRef] [PubMed]
5. Stolzenburg, J.-U.; Arthanareeswaran, V.K.A.; Dietel, A.; Franz, T.; Liatsikos, E.; Kyriazis, I.; Ganzer, R.; Yaney, K.; Do, H.M. Four-Point Peritoneal Flap Fixation in Preventing Lymphocele Formation Following Radical Prostatectomy. *Eur. Urol. Oncol.* **2018**, *1*, 443–448. [CrossRef]
6. Lebeis, C.; Canes, D.; Sorcini, A.; Moinzadeh, A. Novel Technique Prevents Lymphoceles after Transperitoneal Robotic-Assisted Pelvic Lymph Node Dissection: Peritoneal Flap Interposition. *Urology* **2015**, *85*, 1505–1509. [CrossRef]
7. Gloger, S.; Ubrig, B.; Boy, A.; Leyh-Bannurah, S.-R.; Siemer, S.; Arndt, M.; Stolzenburg, J.-U.; Franz, T.; Oelke, M.; Witt, J.H. Bilateral Peritoneal Flaps Reduce Incidence and Complications of Lymphoceles after Robotic Radical Prostatectomy with Pelvic Lymph Node Dissection—Results of the Prospective Randomized Multicenter Trial ProLy. *J. Urol.* **2022**, *208*, 333–340. [CrossRef]
8. Novara, G.; Ficarra, V.; Rosen, R.C.; Artibani, W.; Costello, A.; Eastham, J.A.; Graefen, M.; Guazzoni, G.; Shariat, S.F.; Stolzenburg, J.U.; et al. Systematic Review and Meta-Analysis of Perioperative Outcomes and Complications after Robot-Assisted Radical Prostatectomy. *Eur. Urol.* **2012**, *62*, 431–452. [CrossRef]
9. Heers, H.; Laumeier, T.; Olbert, P.J.; Hofmann, R.; Hegele, A. Lymphoceles Post-Radical Retropubic Prostatectomy: A Retrospective Evaluation of Epidemiology, Risk Factors and Outcome. *Urol. Int.* **2015**, *95*, 400–405. [CrossRef]
10. Magistro, G.; Tuong-Linh Le, D.; Westhofen, T.; Buchner, A.; Schlenker, B.; Becker, A.; Stief, C.G. Occurrence of Symptomatic Lymphocele after Open and Robot-Assisted Radical Prostatectomy. *Cent. Eur. J. Urol.* **2021**, *74*, 341–347.
11. Tsaur, I.; Thomas, C. Risk Factors, Complications and Management of Lymphocele Formation after Radical Prostatectomy: A Mini-Review. *Int. J. Urol.* **2019**, *26*, 711–716. [CrossRef] [PubMed]
12. Thomas, C.; Ziewers, S.; Thomas, A.; Dotzauer, R.; Bartsch, G.; Haferkamp, A.; Tsaur, I. Development of Symptomatic Lymphoceles after Radical Prostatectomy and Pelvic Lymph Node Dissection Is Independent of Surgical Approach: A Single-Center Analysis. *Int. Urol. Nephrol.* **2019**, *51*, 633–640. [CrossRef]
13. Khoder, W.Y.; Trottmann, M.; Buchner, A.; Stuber, A.; Hoffmann, S.; Stief, C.G.; Becker, A.J. Risk Factors for Pelvic Lymphoceles Post-Radical Prostatectomy. *Int. J. Urol.* **2011**, *18*, 638–643. [CrossRef] [PubMed]
14. Motterle, G.; Morlacco, A.; Zanovello, N.; Ahmed, M.E.; Zattoni, F.; Karnes, R.J.; Dal Moro, F. Surgical Strategies for Lymphocele Prevention in Minimally Invasive Radical Prostatectomy and Lymph Node Dissection: A Systematic Review. *J. Endourol.* **2020**, *34*, 113–120. [CrossRef] [PubMed]
15. Kim, W.T.; Ham, W.S.; Koo, K.C.; Choi, Y.D. Efficacy of Octreotide for Management of Lymphorrhea after Pelvic Lymph Node Dissection in Radical Prostatectomy. *Urology* **2010**, *76*, 398–401. [CrossRef]
16. Abaza, R.; Henderson, S.J.; Martinez, O. Robotic Vessel Sealer Device for Lymphocele Prevention after Pelvic Lymphadenectomy: Results of a Randomized Trial. *J. Laparoendosc. Adv. Surg. Tech. A* **2021**, *32*, 721–726. [CrossRef]
17. Yuh, B.E.; Ruel, N.H.; Mejia, R.; Novara, G.; Wilson, T.G. Standardized Comparison of Robot-Assisted Limited and Extended Pelvic Lymphadenectomy for Prostate Cancer. *BJU Int.* **2013**, *112*, 81–88. [CrossRef] [PubMed]
18. Suardi, N.; Larcher, A.; Haese, A.; Ficarra, V.; Govorov, A.; Buffi, N.M.; Walz, J.; Rocco, B.; Borghesi, M.; Steuber, T.; et al. Indication for and Extension of Pelvic Lymph Node Dissection during Robot-Assisted Radical Prostatectomy: An Analysis of Five European Institutions. *Eur. Urol.* **2014**, *66*, 635–643. [CrossRef] [PubMed]
19. Lee, M.; Lee, Z.; Eun, D.D. Utilization of a Peritoneal Interposition Flap to Prevent Symptomatic Lymphoceles after Robotic Radical Prostatectomy and Bilateral Pelvic Lymph Node Dissection. *J. Endourol.* **2020**, *34*, 821–827. [CrossRef] [PubMed]
20. Student, V.; Tudos, Z.; Studentova, Z.; Cesak, O.; Studentova, H.; Repa, V.; Purova, D. Effect of Peritoneal Fixation (PerFix) on Lymphocele Formation in Robot-Assisted Radical Prostatectomy with Pelvic Lymphadenectomy: Results of a Randomized Prospective Trial. *Eur. Urol.* **2023**, *83*, 154–162. [CrossRef]

21. Deutsch, S.; Hadaschik, B.; Lebentrau, S.; Ubrig, B.; Burger, M.; May, M. Clinical Importance of a Peritoneal Interposition Flap to Prevent Symptomatic Lymphoceles after Robot-Assisted Radical Prostatectomy and Pelvic Lymph Node Dissection: A Systematic Review and Meta-Analysis. *Urol. Int.* **2022**, *106*, 28–34. [CrossRef] [PubMed]
22. Bründl, J.; Lenart, S.; Stojanoski, G.; Gilfrich, C.; Rosenhammer, B.; Stolzlechner, M.; Ponholzer, A.; Dreissig, C.; Weikert, S.; Burger, M.; et al. Peritoneal Flap in Robot-Assisted Radical Prostatectomy. *Dtsch. Aerzteblatt Online* **2020**, *117*, 243–250. [CrossRef]
23. Capitanio, U.; Pellucchi, F.; Gallina, A.; Briganti, A.; Suardi, N.; Salonia, A.; Abdollah, F.; Di Trapani, E.; Jeldres, C.; Cestari, A.; et al. How Can We Predict Lymphorrhoea and Clinically Significant Lymphocoeles after Radical Prostatectomy and Pelvic Lymphadenectomy? Clinical Implications. *BJU Int.* **2011**, *107*, 1095–1101. [CrossRef] [PubMed]
24. Naselli, A.; Andreatta, R.; Introini, C.; Fontana, V.; Puppo, P. Predictors of Symptomatic Lymphocele after Lymph Node Excision and Radical Prostatectomy. *Urology* **2010**, *75*, 630–635. [CrossRef]
25. Goßler, C.; May, M.; Breyer, J.; Stojanoski, G.; Weikert, S.; Lenart, S.; Ponholzer, A.; Dreissig, C.; Burger, M.; Gilfrich, C.; et al. High BMI, Aggressive Tumours and Long Console Time Are Independent Predictive Factors for Symptomatic Lymphocele Formation after Robot-Assisted Radical Prostatectomy and Pelvic Lymph Node Dissection. *Urol. Int.* **2021**, *105*, 453–459. [CrossRef] [PubMed]
26. Sforza, S.; Tellini, R.; Grosso, A.A.; Zaccaro, C.; Viola, L.; Di Maida, F.; Mari, A.; Carini, M.; Minervini, A.; Masieri, L. Can We Predict the Development of Symptomatic Lymphocele Following Robot-Assisted Radical Prostatectomy and Lymph Node Dissection? Results from a Tertiary Referral Centre. *Scand. J. Urol.* **2020**, *54*, 328–333. [CrossRef] [PubMed]
27. Goßler, C.; May, M.; Rosenhammer, B.; Breyer, J.; Stojanoski, G.; Weikert, S.; Lenart, S.; Ponholzer, A.; Dreissig, C.; Burger, M.; et al. Obesity Leads to a Higher Rate of Positive Surgical Margins in the Context of Robot-Assisted Radical Prostatectomy. Results of a Prospective Multicenter Study. *Cent. Eur. J. Urol.* **2020**, *73*, 457. [CrossRef]
28. Nishimura, S.; Manabe, I.; Nagai, R. Adipose Tissue Inflammation in Obesity and Metabolic Syndrome. *Discov. Med.* **2009**, *8*, 55–60.
29. Porcaro, A.B.; Sebben, M.; Tafuri, A.; de Luyk, N.; Corsi, P.; Processali, T.; Pirozzi, M.; Rizzetto, R.; Amigoni, N.; Mattevi, D.; et al. Body Mass Index Is an Independent Predictor of Clavien-Dindo Grade 3 Complications in Patients Undergoing Robot Assisted Radical Prostatectomy with Extensive Pelvic Lymph Node Dissection. *J. Robot. Surg.* **2019**, *13*, 83–89. [CrossRef]
30. Mundhenk, J.; Hennenlotter, J.; Alloussi, S.; Selbherr, D.; Martzog, J.C.; Todenhöfer, T.; Kruck, S.; Schwentner, C.; Stenzl, A.; Schilling, D. Influence of Body Mass Index, Surgical Approach and Lymphadenectomy on the Development of Symptomatic Lymphoceles after Radical Prostatectomy. *Urol. Int.* **2013**, *90*, 270–276. [CrossRef]
31. Lee, J.Y.; Diaz, R.R.; Cho, K.S.; Yu, H.S.; Chung, J.S.; Ham, W.S.; Choi, Y.D. Lymphocele after Extraperitoneal Robot-Assisted Radical Prostatectomy: A Propensity Score-Matching Study. *Int. J. Urol.* **2013**, *20*, 1169–1176. [CrossRef]
32. Porcaro, A.B.; Rizzetto, R.; Bianchi, A.; Gallina, S.; Serafin, E.; Panunzio, A.; Tafuri, A.; Cerrato, C.; Migliorini, F.; Zecchini Antoniolli, S.; et al. American Society of Anesthesiologists (ASA) Physical Status System Predicts the Risk of Postoperative Clavien–Dindo Complications Greater than One at 90 Days after Robot-Assisted Radical Prostatectomy: Final Results of a Tertiary Referral Center. *J. Robot. Surg.* **2022**, 1–7. [CrossRef]
33. Touijer, K.A.; Sjoberg, D.D.; Benfante, N.; Laudone, V.P.; Ehdaie, B.; Eastham, J.A.; Scardino, P.T.; Vickers, A. Limited versus Extended Pelvic Lymph Node Dissection for Prostate Cancer: A Randomized Clinical Trial. *Eur. Urol. Oncol.* **2021**, *4*, 532–539. [CrossRef] [PubMed]
34. Lestingi, J.F.P.; Guglielmetti, G.B.; Trinh, Q.D.; Coelho, R.F.; Pontes, J.; Bastos, D.A.; Cordeiro, M.D.; Sarkis, A.S.; Faraj, S.F.; Mitre, A.I.; et al. Extended Versus Limited Pelvic Lymph Node Dissection During Radical Prostatectomy for Intermediate- and High-Risk Prostate Cancer: Early Oncological Outcomes from a Randomized Phase 3 Trial. *Eur. Urol.* **2021**, *79*, 595–604. [CrossRef] [PubMed]
35. Cacciamani, G.E.; Maas, M.; Nassiri, N.; Ortega, D.; Gill, K.; Dell'Oglio, P.; Thalmann, G.N.; Heidenreich, A.; Eastham, J.A.; Evans, C.P.; et al. Impact of Pelvic Lymph Node Dissection and Its Extent on Perioperative Morbidity in Patients Undergoing Radical Prostatectomy for Prostate Cancer: A Comprehensive Systematic Review and Meta-Analysis. *Eur. Urol. Oncol.* **2021**, *4*, 134–149. [CrossRef] [PubMed]

cancers

MDPI

rticle

ocal Endoscopic Treatment of Low-Grade Urothelial Tumors in he Upper Urinary Tract—Oncological Outcome of a Consecutive Single-Center Series of 118 Patients

ophie Bislev [1,*], Simone Buchardt Brandt [1,2], Sven Fuglsig [2] and Jørgen Bjerggaard Jensen [1,2]

1 Department of Clinical Medicine, Aarhus University, 8000 Aarhus C, Denmark; simbra@rm.dk (S.B.B.); bjerggaard@skejby.rm.dk (J.B.J.)
2 Department of Urology, Aarhus University Hospital, 8200 Aarhus N, Denmark; svenfugl@rm.dk
* Correspondence: sbislev@gmail.com

Simple Summary: This paper presents the results of our retrospective cohort single-center study. Our findings demonstrate that patients diagnosed with low-grade upper tract urothelial tumors exhibit a high recurrence rate when treated with laser ablation, but a low progression rate. While the overall mortality in this cohort is relatively high, deaths related specifically to upper tract urothelial tumors are low. Importantly, our data indicate that recurrences primarily occur within the first few years after diagnosis. Thus, vigilant follow-up during this period proves effective in detecting recurrences. We conclude that laser ablation stands as a safe and less invasive alternative to radical nephroureterectomy.

Abstract: Background: Upper urinary tract urothelial tumors are mostly treated with the use of endoscopic laser ablation. The treatment is recommended when the tumor is low grade and non-invasive. Objective: The aim of the present study was to investigate the oncological outcome of patients treated endoscopically for low-grade (LG) upper tract urothelial carcinoma (UTUC). Methods: One hundred and eighteen consecutive patients with pTa LG UTUC initially treated with laser ablation from 2012–2022 at a single university hospital were included. Patient and tumor characteristics, treatment, and oncological outcomes were retrospectively registered from electronic medical journals. Survival analysis was performed using Kaplan–Meier and Nelson–Aalen plots. Results: The median number of local recurrences was 2 with a median time to first recurrence of 5 months (IQR: 2–46). The 2-year share of patients having no recurrence was 28.8%. The risk of recurrence was highest within the first 3 years following initial treatment. Two-year survival function with no progression and preserved renal unit was 67.9%. The two-year overall survival (OS) and disease-specific survival (DSS) were 84.2% and 97.1%. The 5-year OS and DSS were 59.1% and 94.1%. The median follow-up time for OS was 36 months (IQR: 20.3–58.8). Conclusions: In the patient series, we found that the risk of recurrence following laser ablation of LG UTUC was high; however, it was associated with a low risk of progression and high OS and DSS. Therefore, we conclude that treatment with laser ablation in patients with LG UTUC is safe, although frequent follow-up is needed to detect recurrence.

Keywords: laser; ureteroscopy; uteroscopy instrumentation; laparoscopy benign disease; laparoscopy malignant disease

1. Introduction

Upper tract urothelial cancer (UTUC) is a rare type of urothelial cancer with 200 cases a year nationally, and it only represents 15% of all urothelial cancers with the remaining to be found in the urine bladder. The tumor derives from the urothelial and 2/3 are localized in the pelvis and 1/3 in the ureter [1,2].

The European Association of Urology (EAU) guidelines recommend local treatment of upper tract urothelial cancer (UTUC) with laser ablation instead of radical nephroureterectomy (RNU) for patients with low-grade (LG) unifocal tumors or in patients where RNU is contraindicated and local treatment is possible, as RNU is known to be a major operative procedure that includes a number of post-operative and long-term complications [3,4].

Previous studies find no difference in cancer-specific survival (CSS) when comparing local treatment with RNU. These studies include all stages of UTUC. The risk of cancer-specific death was higher in patients with high-grade (HG) UTUC treated locally, and the overall survival (OS) was better in patients with LG UTUC treated locally [5–10].

The kidney-sparing treatment includes the risk of local recurrence. Previous studies have found between 68% and 92% of the patients develop a local recurrence, with an average of more than three recurrences pr. patient [7,11,12].

Previous studies either compare kidney-sparing surgery with radical nephroureterectomy in treatment of both LG and HG tumors regarding survival and recurrence. More specific studies with more narrow inclusion criteria regarding tumor stage and tumor grade are needed.

In the present study, we aimed to investigate the long-term outcomes for patients treated with endoscopic kidney-sparing surgery in patients with pTa og pT1 LG UTUC.

2. Methods

2.1. Patient Recruitment

All patients with pTa low grade (LG) and pT1 LG tumor in the upper urinary tract in the period from 2012–2022 in the Central Region Denmark, which has a population of approximately 1.3 million habitants, were included. Patients were identified through the pathology code registered in the regional pathology database by SNOMED codes registered at the time of pathology examination [13]. The patients were treated in two different public regional hospitals each with their own pathology department.

Individual patient data were obtained retrospectively from electronic patient medical charts. The creatinine clearance was calculated from creatinine level, gender, height, and weight using the Cockcroft–Gault equation [14]. Comorbidities were registered as the Charlson Comorbidity Index [15]. The size of the initial tumor was found either in the CT-scan description or in the surgical note.

All data were collected and managed using REDCap electronic data capture tools version 14.5.16 hosted at the Institute of Clinical Medicine, Health, Aarhus University [16].

2.2. Diagnosis and Treatment Plan

All patients with suspected tumor of the upper urinary tract underwent ureterorenoscopy (URS) with biopsy, unless nephroureterectomy was indicated already or metastases were identified at the time of diagnosis. If the tumor was papillary with no suspicion of invasion, it was most often treated during the same procedure with laser ablation. The laser used was an Olympus Soltive Thulium laser (Tokyo, Japan) with a 150 nm fiber. After the first local treatment, patients with Ta LG tumor underwent a 4-month follow-up control with URS. In cases of no local recurrence, new URS was performed after additional 4 and 8 months and hereafter yearly control CT-urography for three years. Cystoscopy to detect bladder recurrence was performed at all follow-up visits. In patients where local treatment was chosen due to other indications than Ta LG, the follow-up was based on an individual evaluation [2,5,17].

2.3. Statistical Analysis and Outcomes

The Nelson–Aalen plot was used to illustrate the cumulative hazard of getting first local recurrence. A Kaplan–Meier curve was constructed with the same data to illustrate the time in which the local recurrence occurred after diagnosis.

Progression was defined as a progression from pTa LG and included pTa HG. The event was either death, pathological progression to higher stage, or RNU.

Progression-free survival, OS, and CSS were analyzed using Kaplan–Meier curves with standard deviation of the median and interquartile range (IQR). Follow-up time was defined as time from histology verified diagnosis to death or the date of last data entry. Death was noted as either UTUC specific or other cause of death.

The statistical analysis was performed in Microsoft Excel version 16.72 using XLSTAT free trial version.

2.4. Ethical Approvement

The study was approved by the Central Denmark Region Committees on Health Research Ethics (approval ID: 1-45-70-36-23). Signed consent was waived from our ethical committee in patients not alive at the time of data collection, whereas written informed consent was obtained from all living participants involved.

3. Results

3.1. Patient Characteristics

A total of 324 patients fulfilled the pathological SNOMED code criteria for LG NMIBC. Of these, 206 patients were excluded from further analysis for various reasons (Figure 1). This resulted in 118 patients with LG UTUC who underwent initial endoscopic local treatment (Table 1).

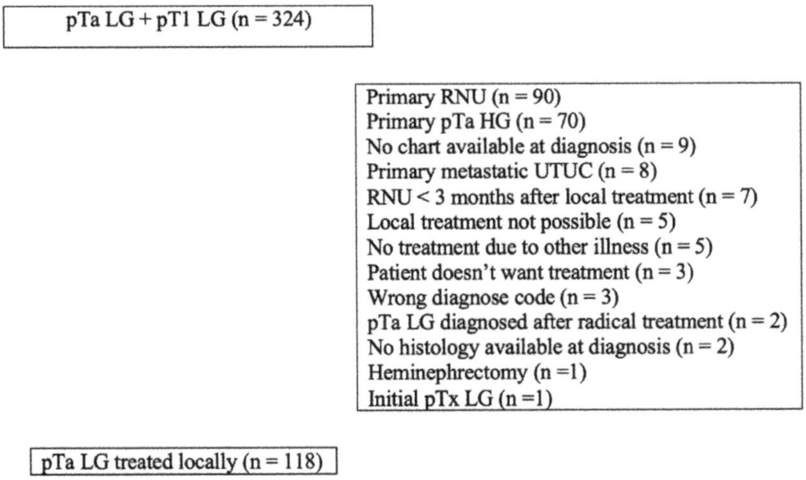

Figure 1. Flow chart showing the inclusion and exclusion of patients.

Table 1. Patient demographic and characteristics and information regarding status at diagnosis and tumor information. N = number, ASA = severe systematic disease, LG = low grade, HG = high grade, NA = not available, RNU = radical nephroureterectomy.

Sex (male/female), n (%)	82 (69.5)/36 (30.5)
Age (years), median (IQR)	75 (69–81)
Body mass index (kg/m^2), median (IQR)	26 (23–28)
No BMI available, n	24
ASA grade, n (%)	
1	8 (6.8)
2	61 (51.7)
3	46 (39.0)
4	2 (1.7)
5	0 (0.0)
NA	1 (0.8)

Table 1. *Cont.*

Charlsons Comorbidity Index, n (%)	
1	26 (26.5)
2	28 (28.6)
3	22 (21.4)
4–5	12 (12.2)
6–7	8 (8.2)
8–9	3 (3.1)
Smoking, n (%)	
Never	42 (35.6)
Former	28 (24.6)
Present	44 (37.3)
NA	3 (2.5)
History of bladder tumors (yes/no), n (%)	40 (35.6)/78 (64.4)
Treatment with cystectomy (yes/no), n (%)	5 (12.5)/35 (87.5)
Former contralateral RNU (yes/no), n (%)	8 (6.8)/110 (93.2)
Diagnosis characteristics	
Hydronephrosis, n (%)	
Yes	23 (19.5)
No	92 (78.0)
NA	3 (25)
Creatinine (μmol/L), median (IQR)	86.5 (73–108)
Creatinine clearance (μmol/L), median (IQR)	63.0 (43.9–79.8)
Number of tumors, n (%)	
1	95 (80.5)
2	18 (15.3)
>2	3 (2.5)
NA	2 (1.7)
Location of tumor, n (%)	
Right	60 (50.8)
Left	54 (45.8)
Bilateral	4 (3.4)
Tumor stage, n (%)	
pTa LG	116 (98.3)
pT1 LG	0 (0.0)
pTis LG	2 (1.7)
Size of largest tumor (mm), median (IQR)	15 (10–20)
Urine cytology at diagnosis n (%)	
LG	78 (66.1)
HG	4 (3.4)
NA	36 (30.5)
JJ-catheter following procedure (yes/no), n (%)	113 (95.8)/5 (4.2)
Acute re-hospitalized within 90 days after procedure (yes/no), n (%)	21 (17.8)/97 (82.2)

3.2. Local Recurrence

The median time from diagnosis to first local recurrence was 5 months (IQR: 2–46). The cumulative HR of getting local recurrence is illustrated in Figure 2. The total follow-up time was 122 months (10.2 years) and the cumulative hazard at this point was 2.0 (IQR: 0.9–3.0) (SE = 0.54). At 12 months (1 year), the HR was 1.0 (SE = 0.13).

One year after initial treatment, 33.8% (SE = 0.045) were local recurrence free (Figure 3). The 2-year RFS was 28.8% (SE = 0.045).

Recurrence characteristics are shown in Table 2.

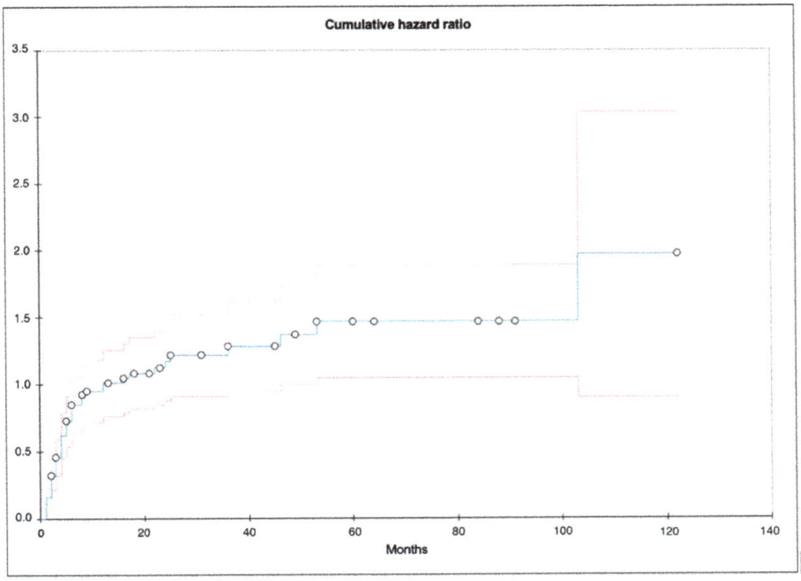

Figure 2. Nilsson–Aalen plot illustrating the hazard ratio of getting a local recurrence after diagnosis. Blue curve = median hazard, upper red curve = 75% quantile, lower red curve = 25% quantile, white spots = event or censored.

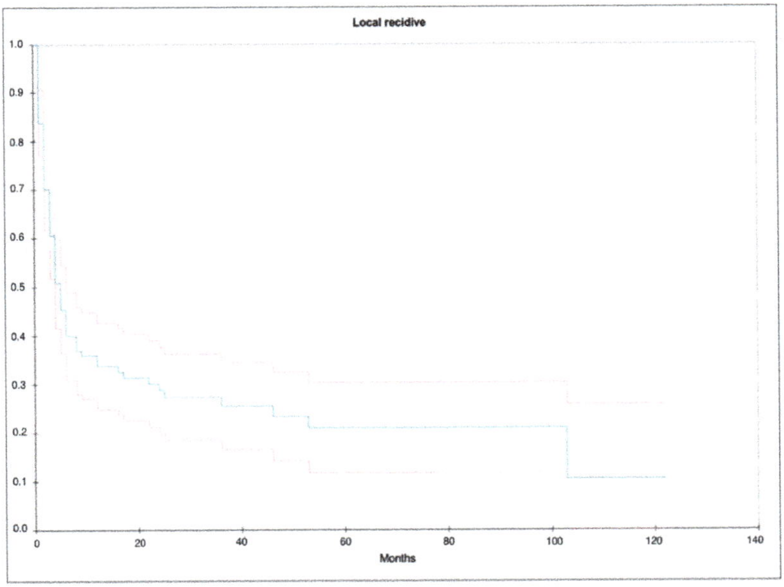

Figure 3. Kaplan–Meier curve illustrating the local recurrence distribution from diagnosis to first local recurrence. Blue curve = median, upper red curve = 75% quantile, lower red curve = 25% quantile.

Table 2. Recurrence information. n = number, BCG = bacille Calmette-Guerin.

Recurrence	
Follow-up duration (months), median (IQR)	36.0 (20.3–58.8)
Local recurrence in upper urinary tract (yes/no), n (%)	83 (69.3)/35 (29.7)
Local recurrence with progression, n (%)	20 (24.1)
Treatment with mitomycin C, n (%)	8 (9.6)
Treatment with BCG, n (%)	5 (6.0)
Recurrence in the contralateral urinary tract, n (%)	10 (12.0)
Recurrence, n (%)	
In bladder	52 (44.1)
Metastatic	5 (4.2)
Number of recurrence pr. Patient, median (IQR)	2 (1–5)
Time to first recurrence (months), median (IQR)	5 (2–46)

3.3. *Progression*

In the present study, 20 out of the 118 patients had local recurrence with progression, and of those, 8 proceeded to RNU. In total, 20 of the 118 patients had salvage RNU (Table 3). The median survival time with no progression or RNU was 48 months (2 years). The 2-year progression and RNU-free survival distribution was 67.9% (SE = 0.044) and the 5-year progression and RNU-free survival was 44.5% (SE = 0.054). The survival distribution is illustrated in Figure 4. The median follow-up time was 26 months (IQR: 11–53).

Table 3. Outcome information. n = number.

Initial pTa LG, n (%)	118 (100)
Salvage nephroureterectomy, n (%)	20 (16.9)
Death, n (%)	42 (35.6)
Death from other cause, n (%)	37 (31.4)
UTUC-specific death (yes/no), n (%)	5 (4.2)

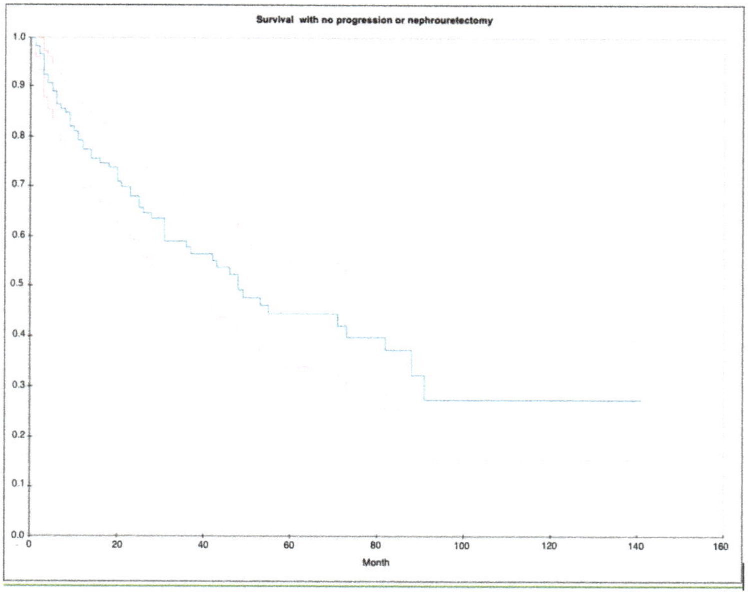

Figure 4. Kaplan–Meier curve illustrating the survival distribution of surviving with no progression and no nephroureterectomy. Blue curve = median, upper red curve = 75% quantile, lower red curve = 25% quantile.

3.4. Long Term Survival

The median follow-up time was 36.0 months (IQR: 20.3–58.8). Figure 5A illustrates the OS and the CSS. The OS after a total follow-up of 141 months (11.8 years) was 38.9% (SE = 0.074). The 2-year OS was 84.2% (SE = 0.035) and the 5-year OS was 59.1% (SE = 0.057). The median OS time was 88 months (7.3 years) after diagnosis.

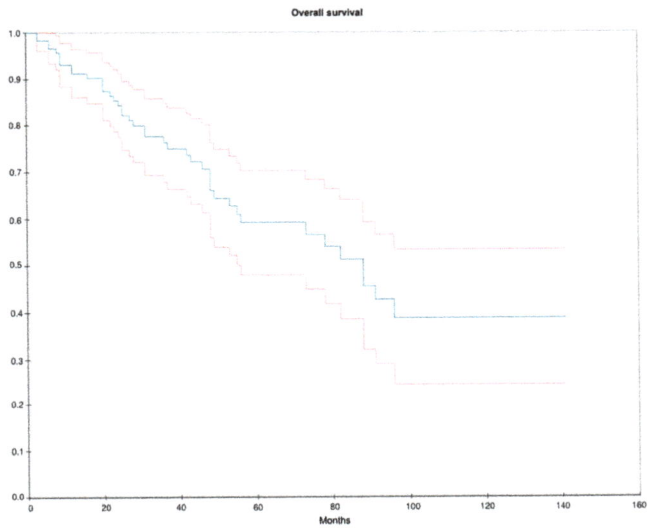

(A)

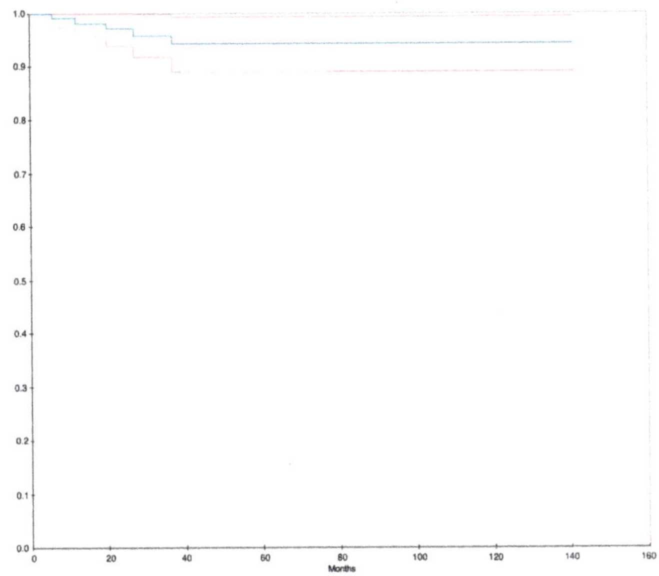

(B)

Figure 5. (**A**): Kaplan–Meier curve illustrating overall survival from diagnosis to death or date of data collection. Blue curve = median, upper red curve = 75% quantile, lower red curve = 25% quantile. (**B**): Kaplan–Meier curve illustrating disease-specific survival from diagnosis to death from disease or data collection. Blue curve = median, upper red curve = 75% quantile, lower red curve = 25% quantile.

The DSS was 94.1% (SE = 0.026) at end of follow-up (141 months); no patients had a disease-specific death after 36 months of follow-up, illustrated in Figure 5B. The 2-year DSS was 97.1% (SE = 0.017). The median disease-specific mortality time was 20 months (IQR: 12–27).

4. Discussion

In the present patient series, we found that the local recurrence rate following local laser ablation in LG UTUC was high. However, we also found that risk of progression was low, and that the CSS was clearly higher than the OS. Thus, we found that the mortality is predominantly related to other causes than the urothelial tumor following local laser ablation, indicating that it is a safe procedure in selected patients.

Seisen et al. found no difference in CSS when comparing local treatment with RNU in a systematic review from 2016 [5]. They defined local treatment as both segmental ureterectomy and endoscopic procedures. In five of the included twenty-two studies from the meta-analysis, endoscopic treatment was compared with RNU. Here, no significant difference in 5-year and 10-year CSS was found between endoscopic treatment and RNU. The studies included all T-stages of UTUC. They found that the risk of cancer-specific death was higher in patients with HG UTUC who received endoscopic treatment, whereas the OS was significantly better in the patients with LG UTUC undergoing endoscopic treatment. These findings are contradicted in a retrospective study by Kim et al., who found that OS and CSS after 24 months were similar when treated endoscopically compared with RNU, but after 24 months, the OS and CSS were lower for patients treated endoscopically. However, the group of endoscopically treated patients had a large heterogeneity since comorbidities were more frequent and the patients were older, for which the investigators did not adjust for [6].

The OS found in this study is the OS of patients with a diagnosis of LG UTUC treated with laser ablation initially. The OS is relatively low and could be due to the high mean age at diagnosis. Furthermore, this study finds a higher recurrence rate than other similar studies. This could be due to more patients being selected for local treatment over RNU in this study than in other studies [7,11,12]. Another bias that could have underestimated the OS in the present study is that potential heredity was not obtained from the patients. A study shows that 5.2% of the patients having UTUC had confirmed Lynch syndrome, and these patients have higher risk of specific cancer types [18].

The local recurrence and median time from diagnosis to first local recurrence are lower in the present study compared to those reported in Shenhar et al., where 92% had local recurrence with an average of 3.2 recurrence pr. patient. This could be due to the difference in inclusion criteria, where the patients in the present study had lower stages of tumors. In the present study, 24.1% underwent salvage RNU after initial local treatment, compared to only 17% reported by Shenhar et al., despite the patients in the present study having lower stages. However, this discrepancy could reflect the differences in national guidelines of when to perform RNU initially [11].

The risk of local recurrence following endoscopic treatment of UTUC is important to consider when offering endoscopic treatment. We found that the risk of local recurrence was highest within the first 18 months following initial treatment. The currently recommended control program after diagnosis recommends follow-up for a minimum of 5 years but often lifelong [3]. After 5 years, the cumulative incidence increases from 1.5 to 2.0 in our present series; however, this is based on only one patient who had a first local recurrence after 5 years. This could indicate that the current control program is sufficient for diagnosing local recurrence and could be terminated following a 5-year recurrence-free interval and only be undergoing new investigations in case of symptoms [3]. The current national guidelines of treatment of urothelial tumors in the upper urinary tract are based on retrospective studies, where local treatment is compared with RNU or studies where the outcomes of local treatment are illustrated. In these studies, no significant difference was found in oncological outcomes [19].

The EAU recommends RNU in cases of HG UTUC [17]. Studies have found the disease-free OS to be between 66% and 71% and the 5-year DSS to be between 72% and 75% [20,21]. The studies only include HG UTUC. Compared to this study, especially the DSS is much lower than the DSS found in the present study. The outcomes of these studies are difficult to compare directly, as the patient groups included are not comparable due the difference in disease severity. If compared, endoscopic treatment is related to a better CSS than RNU, but a large bias in comparison is the patient groups, as HG UTUC is known to have a lower CSS than LG UTUC [22,23]. Other kidney-sparing treatment methods for UTUC located in the ureter are segmental ureteral resection or percutaneous access. This is recommended for LG UTUC that cannot be removed endoscopically [17,24]. Studies show no significant difference in short-term outcomes comparing RNU and segmental ureteral resection, but these methods are used less due to improved endoscopic tools [24–26]. A study investigating the oncological outcome after percutaneous endoscopic resection showed a 5-year DSS of 79.5%, which is lower than that found in the present series, indicating that the endoscopic procedure is associated with higher survival. The bias of this study was the low number of included patients (n = 40) [27].

The present study is limited by the retrospective design and the absence of continuous monitoring throughout the follow-up period from the patient's last visit to the department until data entry; however, the risk of local recurrence hereafter is low. Furthermore, the data were collected from the regional chart system; however, not all data were accessible and were simply not registered. An important factor that lacked in a series of patients in the present study was the size of the initial tumor. The present study stands out from other studies in the current literature due to the large number of patients included [2,5,7].

Retrospectively, a series of data was not obtained from the patients, which could have been interesting to include in the analysis. An important factor that was missed was which of the patients had previous bladder cancer, as bladder cancer is known as a risk factor of getting UTUC [28,29]. This could underestimate the OS, as 30 patients from this study had a history of bladder cancer. A subgroup analysis should have been performed to exclude the 40 patients who had a history of bladder cancer. Another factor that we missed was the marital status of the patients, as this could have had an impact on the effect of the treatment pattern.

Although the number of patients in this study is relatively large, if a larger cohort size is desired, the same kind of study could be conducted in 5–10 years. The next step in this research could be to conduct a study where the two treatment methods, local treatment of RNU, for these types of patients could be compared to see if the patients who undergo RNU have better outcomes than patients treated locally. Another outcome parameter in this kind of study could be the development of kidney function after treatment alongside survival distributions. Furthermore, the effect of treatment with BCG or mitomycin C was not investigated in this study. In further research, it could be interesting to determine if it has the same effect as in treatment of bladder tumors [30].

5. Conclusions

In conclusion, patients diagnosed with LG UTUC tumors have a high local recurrence rate but a low rate of progression. We find that close post-operative follow-up for the first few years is indicated to detect early local recurrences. The overall mortality rate is high in this cohort; however, only a small fraction of deaths is related to UTUC after initial local treatment. We find that local ablation is a safe and less invasive alternative to up-front RNU, which is associated with high DSS for treatment of UTUC.

Author Contributions: S.B.: conceptualization, methodology, software, formal analysis, investigation, data curation, writing—original draft, visualization. S.B.B.: conceptualization, methodology, validation, formal analysis, writing—review and editing, supervision. S.F.: conceptualization, validation, writing—review and editing. J.B.J.: conceptualization, methodology, validation, resources, writing—review and editing, supervision. All authors have read and agreed to the published version of the manuscript.

Funding: This research received no external funding.

Institutional Review Board Statement: The study was approved 5 April 2023 by the Central Denmark Region Committees on Health Research Ethics (approval ID: 1-45-70-36-23).

Informed Consent Statement: Signed consent was waived from our ethical committee in patients not alive at the time of data collection whereas written informed consent was obtained from all living participants involved.

Data Availability Statement: The datasets presented in this article are not readily available because of Danish law (general data protection regulation (GDPR)) regarding personal information that says this information cannot be handed out without legal permission.

Conflicts of Interest: J.B.J reports grants and personal fees from Photocure ASA, Olympus, Ferring, Cepheid, Nucleix, medac, Pfizer, MSD, Astellas, Astra-Zenica, Ambu, and IntuitiveSurgery, and nonfinancial support from Roche outside the submitted work. The remaining authors have no conflicts of interest to report.

Abbreviations

LG	Low grade
UTUC	Upper tract urothelial cancer
EAU	European Association of Urology
OS	Overall survival
DSS	Disease-specific survival
CSS	Cancer-specific survival
HG	High grade
URS	Ureterorenoscopy
IQR	Interquartile range
SE	Standard error
RNU	Radical nephroureterectomy

References

1. Borre, M.; Sengeløv, L.; Bonfils, P.; Bojer, D. Uroteliale tTumorer i de Øvre Urinveje. Lægehåndbogen. 2022. Available online: https://www.sundhed.dk/sundhedsfaglig/laegehaandbogen/nyrer-og-urinveje/tilstande-og-sygdomme/urinvejssygdomme/uroteliale-tumorer-i-oevre-urinveje/ (accessed on 17 March 2023).
2. Dansk BlæreCancer Gruppe. *Behandling af Uroteliale Tumorer i Øvre Urinvej*; Kliniske Retningslinjer i Kræft: Aarhus, Denmark, 2022.
3. Rouprêt, M.; Gontero, P.; Birtle, A.; Compérat, E.M.; Dominguez-Escrig, J.L.; Liedberg, F.; Mariappan, P.; Masson-Lecomte, A.; Mostafid, A.H.; van Rhijn, B.W.G.; et al. *EAU Guidelines on Upper Urinary Tract Urothelial Cell Carcinoma*; European Association of Urology: Arnhem, The Netherlands, 2023.
4. Raman, J.; Shore, N.D. Management of Low-grade Upper Tract Urothelial Carcinoma: An Unmet Need. *Rev. Urol.* **2020**, *22*, 1–8. [PubMed]
5. Seisen, T.; Peyronnet, B.; Dominguez-Escrig, J.L.; Bruins, H.M.; Yuan, C.Y.; Babjuk, M.; Böhle, A.; Burger, M.; Compérat, E.M.; Cowan, N.C.; et al. Oncologic Outcomes of Kidney-sparing Surgery Versus Radical Nephroureterectomy for Upper Tract Urothelial Carcinoma: A Systematic Review by the EAU Non-muscle Invasive Bladder Cancer Guidelines Panel. *Eur. Urol.* **2016**, *70*, 1052–1068. [CrossRef] [PubMed]
6. Vemana, G.; Kim, E.H.; Bhayani, S.B.; Vetter, J.M.; Strope, S.A. Survival Comparison Between Endoscopic and Surgical Management for Patients With Upper Tract Urothelial Cancer: A Matched Propensity Score Analysis Using Surveillance, Epidemiology and End Results-Medicare Data. *Urology* **2016**, *95*, 115–120. [CrossRef] [PubMed]
7. Cutress, M.L.; Stewart, G.D.; Wells-Cole, S.; Phipps, S.; Thomas, B.G.; Tolley, D.A. Long-term endoscopic management of upper tract urothelial carcinoma: 20-year single-centre experience. *BJU Int.* **2012**, *110*, 1608–1617. [CrossRef]
8. Hasan, M.N.; Rouprêt, M.; Keeley, F.; Cracco, C.; Jones, R.; Straub, M.; Traxer, O.; Osther, P.J.S.; Brehmer, M. Consultation on UTUC, Stockholm 2018 aspects of risk stratification: Long-term results and follow-up. *World J. Urol.* **2019**, *37*, 2289–2296. [CrossRef]
9. Kawada, T.; Laukhtina, E.; Araki, M.; Shariat, S.F. Reply to Kun-Peng Li, Shun Wan, Chen-Yang Wang, and Li Yang's Letter to the Editor re: Tatsushi Kawada, Ekaterina Laukhtina, Fahad Quhal, et al. Oncologic and Safety Outcomes for Endoscopic Surgery Versus Radical Nephroureterectomy for Upper Tract Urothelial Carcinoma: An Updated Systematic Review and Meta-analysis. Eur Urol Focus 2023;9:236-40. *Eur. Urol. Focus* **2024**, *10*, 492.
10. Rouprêt, M. Conservative management of urothelial carcinomas of the upper urinary tract. *Prog. Urol.* **2012**, *22*, 861–866. [CrossRef]

11. Shenhar, C.; Veredgorn, Y.; Bulis, S.; Aviv, T.; Darawsha, A.E.; Gilad, R.; Baniel, J.; Ehrlich, Y.; Lifshitz, D. Endoscopic Management of Low-Grade Upper Tract Urothelial Carcinoma: Characterizing the Long-term Burden of Care in Comparison to Radical Nephroureterectomy. *Urology* **2022**, *159*, 152–159. [CrossRef]
12. Milojevic, B.; Dzamic, Z.; Kajmakovic, B.; Milenkovic Petronic, D.; Sipetic Grujicic, S. Urothelial carcinoma: Recurrence and risk factors. *JBUON* **2015**, *20*, 391–398.
13. Hansen, E.; Larsson, H.; Nørgaard, M.; Thind, P.; Jensen, J.B. The Danish Bladder Cancer Database. *Clin. Epidemiol.* **2016**, *8*, 439–443. [CrossRef]
14. Cockcroft, D.W.; Gault, M.H. Prediction of creatinine clearance from serum creatinine. *Nephron* **1976**, *16*, 31–41. [CrossRef] [PubMed]
15. Charlson, M.E.; Carrozzino, D.; Guidi, J.; Patierno, C. Charlson Comorbidity Index: A Critical Review of Clinimetric Properties. *Psychother. Psychosom.* **2022**, *91*, 8–35. [CrossRef] [PubMed]
16. Harris, P.A.; Taylor, R.; Thielke, R.; Payne, J.; Gonzalez, N.; Conde, J.G. Research electronic data capture (REDCap)—A metadata-driven methodology and workflow process for providing translational research informatics support. *J. Biomed. Inform.* **2009**, *42*, 377–381. [CrossRef] [PubMed]
17. Masson-Lecomte, A.; Gontero, P.; Birtle, A.; Compérat, E.; Dominguez Escrig, J.L.; Liedberg, F.; Mariappan, P.; Mostafid, A.H.; van Rhijn, B.W.G.; Seisen, T.; et al. *EAU Guidelines on Urothelial Carcinoma of the Upper Urinary Tract (UTUCs)*; European Association of Urology: Arnhem, The Netherlands, 2024.
18. Metcalfe, M.J.; Petros, F.G.; Rao, P.; Mork, M.E.; Xiao, L.; Broaddus, R.R.; Matin, S.F. Universal Point of Care Testing for Lynch Syndrome in Patients with Upper Tract Urothelial Carcinoma. *J. Urol.* **2018**, *199*, 60–65. [CrossRef]
19. Chen, Y.; Xu, C.; Mou, Z.; Hu, Y.; Yang, C.; Hu, J.; Chen, X.; Luo, J.; Zou, L.; Jiang, H. Endoscopic Cryoablation Versus Radical Nephroureterectomy for Upper Tract Urothelial Carcinoma. *Eur. Urol. Oncol.* 2024, *in press*.
20. Adibi, M.; Youssef, R.; Shariat, S.F.; Lotan, Y.; Wood, C.G.; Sagalowsky, A.I.; Zigeuner, R.; Montorsi, F.; Bolenz, C.; Margulis, V. Oncological outcomes after radical nephroureterectomy for upper tract urothelial carcinoma: Comparison over the three decades. *Int. J. Urol.* **2012**, *19*, 1060–1066. [CrossRef]
21. Shigeta, K.; Kikuchi, E.; Abe, T.; Hagiwara, M.; Ogihara, K.; Anno, T.; Umeda, K.; Baba, Y.; Sanjo, T.; Shojo, K.; et al. Long-Term Oncologic Outcomes of Laparoscopic Versus Open Radical Nephroureterectomy for Patients with T3N0M0 Upper Tract Urothelial Carcinoma: A Multicenter Cohort Study with Adjustment by Propensity Score Matching. *Ann. Surg. Oncol.* **2019**, *26*, 3774–3781. [CrossRef]
22. Mori, K.; Janisch, F.; Parizi, M.K.; Mostafaei, H.; Lysenko, I.; Kimura, S.; Enikeev, D.V.; Egawa, S.; Shariat, S.F. Prognostic Value of Variant Histology in Upper Tract Urothelial Carcinoma Treated with Nephroureterectomy: A Systematic Review and Meta-Analysis. *J. Urol.* **2020**, *203*, 1075–1084. [CrossRef]
23. Rink, M.; Robinson, B.D.; Green, D.A.; Cha, E.K.; Hansen, J.; Comploj, E.; Margulis, V.; Raman, J.D.; Ng, C.K.; Remzi, M.; et al. Impact of histological variants on clinical outcomes of patients with upper urinary tract urothelial carcinoma. *J. Urol.* **2012**, *188*, 398–404. [CrossRef]
24. Colin, P.; Ouzzane, A.; Pignot, G.; Ravier, E.; Crouzet, S.; Ariane, M.M.; Audouin, M.; Neuzillet, Y.; Albouy, B.; Hurel, S.; et al. Comparison of oncological outcomes after segmental ureterectomy or radical nephroureterectomy in urothelial carcinomas of the upper urinary tract: Results from a large French multicentre study. *BJU Int.* **2012**, *110*, 1134–1141. [CrossRef]
25. Jeldres, C.; Lughezzani, G.; Sun, M.; Isbarn, H.; Shariat, S.F.; Budaus, L.; Lattouf, J.B.; Widmer, H.; Graefen, M.; Montorsi, F.; et al. Segmental ureterectomy can safely be performed in patients with transitional cell carcinoma of the ureter. *J. Urol.* **2010**, *183*, 1324–1329. [CrossRef]
26. Cutress, M.L.; Stewart, G.D.; Zakikhani, P.; Phipps, S.; Thomas, B.G.; Tolley, D.A. Ureteroscopic and percutaneous management of upper tract urothelial carcinoma (UTUC): Systematic review. *BJU Int.* **2012**, *110*, 614–628. [CrossRef] [PubMed]
27. Rouprêt, M.; Traxer, O.; Tligui, M.; Conort, P.; Chartier-Kastler, E.; Richard, F.; Cussenot, O. Upper urinary tract transitional cell carcinoma: Recurrence rate after percutaneous endoscopic resection. *Eur. Urol.* **2007**, *51*, 709–713; discussion 714. [CrossRef] [PubMed]
28. Kiss, B.; Furrer, M.A.; Wuethrich, P.Y.; Burkhard, F.C.; Thalmann, G.N.; Roth, B. Stenting Prior to Cystectomy is an Independent Risk Factor for Upper Urinary Tract Recurrence. *J. Urol.* **2017**, *198*, 1263–1268. [CrossRef] [PubMed]
29. Sountoulides, P.; Pyrgidis, N.; Brookman-May, S.; Mykoniatis, I.; Karasavvidis, T.; Hatzichristou, D. Does Ureteral Stenting Increase the Risk of Metachronous Upper Tract Urothelial Carcinoma in Patients with Bladder Tumors? A Systematic Review and Meta-analysis. *J. Urol.* **2021**, *205*, 956–966. [CrossRef]
30. Böhle, A.; Bock, P.R. Intravesical bacille Calmette-Guérin versus mitomycin C in superficial bladder cancer: Formal meta-analysis of comparative studies on tumor progression. *Urology* **2004**, *63*, 682–686; discussion 686–687. [CrossRef]

cancers

MDPI

Review

Posterior Retroperitoneal Laparoscopic Adrenalectomy: An Anatomical Essay and Surgical Update

Bogdan Ovidiu Feciche [1,2], Vlad Barbos [2,3,*], Alexandru Big [2], Daniel Porav-Hodade [4], Alin Adrian Cumpanas [5], Silviu Constantin Latcu [3,5], Flavia Zara [6], Alina Cristina Barb [6], Cristina-Stefania Dumitru [6], Talida Georgiana Cut [7,8], Hossam Ismail [9] and Dorin Novacescu [6]

1 Department of Surgical Disciplines, Discipline of Urology, Faculty of Medicine and Pharmacy, University of Oradea, University Street, No. 1, 410087 Oradea, Romania; feciche.bogdanovidiu@didactic.uoradea.ro
2 Department of Urology, Emergency County Hospital Oradea, Gheorghe Doja Street, No. 65, 410169 Oradea, Romania; alex_big_jsd@yahoo.ro
3 Doctoral School, Victor Babes University of Medicine and Pharmacy Timisoara, E. Murgu Square, No. 2, 300041 Timisoara, Romania; silviu.latcu@umft.ro
4 Department of Urology, George Emil Palade University of Medicine, Pharmacy, Sciences and Technology of Targu-Mures, Gh. Marinescu Street, No. 38, 540142 Targu-Mures, Romania; daniel.porav-hodade@umfst.ro
5 Department XV, Discipline of Urology, Victor Babes University of Medicine and Pharmacy Timisoara, E. Murgu Square, No. 2, 300041 Timisoara, Romania; cumpanas.alin@umft.ro
6 Department II of Microscopic Morphology, Victor Babes University of Medicine and Pharmacy Timisoara, E. Murgu Square, No. 2, 300041 Timisoara, Romania; flavia.zara@umft.ro (F.Z.); toma.alina@umft.ro (A.C.B.); cristina-stefania.dumitru@umft.ro (C.-S.D.); novacescu.dorin@umft.ro (D.N.)
7 Department XIII, Discipline of Infectious Diseases, Victor Babes University of Medicine and Pharmacy Timisoara, E. Murgu Square, No. 2, 300041 Timisoara, Romania; talida.cut@umft.ro
8 Center for Ethics in Human Genetic Identifications, Victor Babes University of Medicine and Pharmacy Timisoara, E. Murgu Square, No. 2, 300041 Timisoara, Romania
9 Department of Urology, Lausitz Seeland Teaching Hospital, University of Dresden, Maria-Grollmuß-Straße, No. 10, 02977 Hoyerswerda, Germany; drismailhossam@gmail.com
* Correspondence: vlad.barbos@umft.ro; Tel.: +40-746-848-349

Simple Summary: This paper explores a modern surgical technique called posterior retroperitoneal laparoscopic adrenalectomy (PRLA), which is used to remove the adrenal glands. Unlike traditional open surgery, PRLA uses small incisions in the patient's back, allowing surgeons to access the adrenal glands directly without disturbing other organs in the abdomen. Here, we explain the complex anatomy involved, describe how surgeons perform this procedure step by step, and discuss its benefits and challenges. PRLA can lead to less pain after surgery, shorter hospital stays, and quicker recovery for patients. However, it requires surgeons to have a deep understanding of the body's structure from a different angle than they are used to. This technique is becoming increasingly popular, but it is not suitable for every patient. Our goal is to help surgeons better understand PRLA, potentially improving outcomes for patients who need adrenal gland surgery.

Abstract: Posterior retroperitoneal laparoscopic adrenalectomy (PRLA) has emerged as a revolutionary, minimally invasive technique for adrenal gland surgery, offering significant advantages over traditional open approaches. This narrative review aims to provide a comprehensive update on PRLA, focusing on its anatomical foundations, surgical technique, and clinical implications. We conducted an extensive review of the current literature and surgical practices to elucidate the key aspects of PRLA. The procedure leverages a unique "backdoor" approach, accessing the adrenal glands through the retroperitoneum, which necessitates a thorough understanding of the posterior abdominal wall and retroperitoneal anatomy. Proper patient selection, meticulous surgical planning, and adherence to key technical principles are paramount for successful outcomes. In this paper, the surgical technique is described step by step, emphasizing critical aspects such as patient positioning, trocar placement, and adrenal dissection. PRLA demonstrates reduced postoperative pain, shorter hospital stays, and faster recovery times compared to open surgery, while maintaining comparable oncological outcomes for appropriately selected cases. However, the technique presents unique challenges, including a confined working space and the need for surgeons to adapt to a posterior anatomical perspective. We conclude that PRLA, in the right clinical setting, offers a safe and effective alternative to traditional adrenalectomy approaches. Future research should focus on expanding indications and refining techniques to further improve patient outcomes.

Keywords: adrenal cancer; adrenal gland morphology; suprarenal gland histology; retroperitoneum/retroperitoneal topography; abdominal wall anatomy; surgical anatomy; minimally invasive surgery; trocar placement technique; operative protocol

1. Introduction

The adrenal glands, or suprarenal glands, first described in 1552 by Bartholomaeus Eustachius, were not well understood until the 19th century, when Thomas Addison described adrenal insufficiency [1]. The first successful adrenalectomy was performed in the early 1900s [2], marking the beginning of surgical interventions for adrenal diseases. The adrenal glands, located deep within the upper retroperitoneum, historically necessitated large thoraco-abdominal incisions, either anterior or posterior, for access during open procedures. This approach, while effective, was associated with significant morbidity, including substantial postoperative pain, parietal complications, extended hospital stays, and lengthy recovery periods, as well as higher overall complication rates. Almost a century later, the introduction of minimally invasive techniques marked a turning point in adrenal surgery, offering patients the benefits of reduced morbidity and improved outcomes.

Laparoscopic adrenalectomy (LA) has revolutionized the surgical management of adrenal gland disorders, establishing itself as a superior alternative to traditional open surgery. The development of laparoscopic nephrectomy in 1990 paved the way for minimally invasive techniques that revolutionized the field [3]. The first LA was conducted by Go et al. on 17 January 1992, in Japan [4]. The initial publication on this procedure was authored by Higashihara et al. in July 1992 [5]. Subsequently, Gagner et al. reported their first case in November 1992, having performed it in March of the same year [6]. This pioneering procedure quickly gained traction, with several groups publishing case series that emphasized the considerable advantages of this new approach, including shorter postoperative hospital stays, fewer wound complications, reduced pain, and a faster return to normal daily activities [3].

Subsequently, building upon these early groundbreaking surgical developments, numerous studies have further validated the feasibility and efficacy of LA. Although many of these studies were retrospective and involved relatively small patient cohorts, they consistently demonstrated that LA outperformed open surgery in several key areas. Notably, LA was associated with less intraoperative blood loss, shorter hospitalization intervals, and fewer overall complications [7,8]. Initially, the operative times for LA were longer compared to open surgery. However, as surgical teams gained experience with advanced laparoscopic techniques, particularly adrenalectomy, these times became comparable to those of the open approach [9]. Furthermore, LA required fewer postoperative analgesics and facilitated quicker social reintegration, thus reinforcing its current status as the gold standard for adrenal surgery in most patients.

Early on, the anterior transperitoneal LA quickly gained popularity due to its familiar anatomy, ample working space, and versatility in accessing both adrenal glands, with the caveat of requiring patient repositioning [6]. Over the following decades, the transperitoneal approach became the gold standard for the surgical management of most adrenal disorders, including functional adrenal tumors (such as pheochromocytomas, aldosterone- and cortisol-secreting adenomas, etc.), non-functional tumors with risk of malignancy, and isolated adrenal metastases, provided there is no invasion into surrounding tissues [10–12].

However, the transperitoneal approach has certain limitations that can impact its suitability for some patients. Entering the deep supero-medial retroperitoneal space anteriorly necessitates the mobilization of adjacent organs, such as the liver, spleen, and pancreas, which can be challenging in the presence of adhesions from prior abdominal surgeries. The intraperitoneal insufflation required for transperitoneal laparoscopy can also cause hemodynamic and respiratory changes that may not be well tolerated by some patients, particularly those with cardiopulmonary comorbidities. Furthermore, bilateral adrenalectomy performed transperitoneally requires repositioning the patient during the procedure, prolonging the operative time and increasing the risk of complications [13].

To address these limitations, the posterior retroperitoneal approach to laparoscopic adrenalectomy (PRLA) was developed in the mid-1990s by Mercan et al. [14] and Walz et al. [15]. By accessing the adrenal glands through the posterior abdominal wall, directly into the retroperitoneal space, PRLA avoids the need to enter the peritoneal cavity or mobilize adjacent organs. This results in several advantages, including shorter operative times, reduced operative complexity, less blood loss and postoperative pain, and faster recovery, compared to the transperitoneal approach [15]. Additionally, PRLA allows for bilateral adrenalectomy without the need for patient repositioning, making it an attractive option for patients with bilateral adrenal disease, such as primary pigmented nodular adrenocortical disease or bilateral pheochromocytomas [16]. Moreover, the posterior retroperitoneal approach, due to its unique patient positioning, even allows for simultaneous bilateral adrenalectomy, with two distinct teams, each operating on a different side, at the same time [17].

Notwithstanding its potential benefits, the adoption of PRLA was initially slow due to several factors. The retroperitoneal anatomy is generally less familiar to many surgeons, and the limited working space can make the procedure technically challenging, especially for those with less experience in minimally invasive adrenal surgery. There were also concerns about the learning curve associated with PRLA and the potential for complications, such as bleeding or injury to adjacent vascular structures.

Over time, however, technical refinements and increasing surgeon experience have helped to overcome these challenges and establish PRLA as a safe and effective alternative to the transperitoneal approach. The most significant contributions to the evolution of PRLA came from Walz et al. in the early 2000s [18], who introduced several modifications to the technique, including the use of higher insufflation pressures (20–25 mmHg) to create a larger working space, as well as a standardized approach to adrenal gland dissection. In their seminal series of 560 PRLAs, Walz et al. demonstrated excellent outcomes, with a low rate of major complications (1.3%), high success rate (98.1%), and applicability to a wide range of adrenal pathologies, including pheochromocytomas, aldosterone-/cortisol-secreting adenomas, and adrenal metastases [18]. Subsequently, larger systematic reviews and meta-analyses [19,20] have corroborated the findings of Walz et al. and provided further evidence supporting the aforementioned operative advantages of PRLA over the transperitoneal approach, with comparable outcomes in terms of complications and success rates [20].

This narrative review aims to provide a comprehensive update on the role of PRLA in modern adrenal surgery, focusing on patient selection, indications, contraindications, and technical considerations, while extensively exploring the intricate surgical anatomy of the adrenal glands and discussing critical retroperitoneal topography and abdominal parietal architecture, emphasizing their practical implications for PRLA. By examining the latest evidence and expert opinions, we seek to guide surgical decision-making and optimize outcomes for patients undergoing adrenalectomy. Through this in-depth exploration of surgical anatomy and operative protocols, we hope to equip surgeons with the knowledge and tools necessary to successfully integrate PRLA into their surgical practice and offer their patients the benefits of this innovative approach to adrenal surgery.

2. Adrenalectomy Approach Selection Considerations

As the body of evidence supporting PRLA continues to grow, it has emerged as a valuable option in the armamentarium of minimally invasive adrenal surgery. Its distinct advantages, particularly for patients with bilateral adrenal disease, prior abdominal surgery, or those seeking faster recovery, have solidified its role in the surgical management of adrenal disorders. However, it is crucial for surgeons to have a deep understanding of the indications, contraindications, and technical nuances of PRLA to ensure optimal patient selection and outcomes.

The decision to perform adrenalectomy is based on several factors, primarily categorized into three main indications: First, functional adrenal tumors, regardless of size, generally warrant surgical intervention. These include tumors responsible for primary Cushing's syndrome (hypersecretion of cortisol) and primary Conn's syndrome (hypersecretion of aldosterone), as well as pheochromocytomas (catecholamine-producing tumors) [21]. In some cases, bilateral adrenalectomy may be necessary, particularly in certain forms of Cushing's disease or in multiple endocrine neoplasia (MEN) syndromes [22].

The second category encompasses tumors with suspected or confirmed malignancy. Adrenocortical carcinoma, though rare, presents a significant challenge, with approximately half being non-functional and the remainder secreting various hormones. Malignant pheochromocytomas, accounting for 12–29% of all pheochromocytomas, pose a diagnostic dilemma due to the lack of definitive preoperative imaging or histological criteria for malignancy. Additionally, metastatic tumors in the adrenal glands, commonly in lymphomas or from primary sites such as the lungs, breast, liver, colon, melanomas, and kidneys, may necessitate adrenalectomy [1,22].

The third category involves non-functional tumors with a risk of malignancy, primarily determined by the size of the lesion. A correlation exists between tumor size and malignancy risk, with lesions larger than 6 cm carrying a 25% risk of malignancy [21]. This size-based approach to surgical decision-making has become a crucial factor in the management of incidentally discovered adrenal masses.

Herein, the management of adrenal masses requires a nuanced approach, balancing the risks of malignancy and hormonal dysfunction against the potential morbidity of surgical intervention. While clear guidelines exist for functional tumors and those with high suspicion of malignancy, the management of non-functional incidentalomas remains a subject of ongoing research and debate in the endocrine surgery community [1].

In contemporary practice, the choice between PRLA and other adrenalectomy approaches depends on a careful consideration of patient factors, tumor characteristics, and surgeon experience. A thorough preoperative evaluation, including hormonal testing, high-resolution imaging, and assessment of comorbidities, is essential to guide surgical decision-making [23]. Ultimately, the goal is to select the approach that offers the best balance of safety, efficacy, and patient outcomes.

Advances in radiological imaging have increased the detection of adrenal incidentalomas—adrenal masses $\geq$ 1 cm in diameter discovered incidentally during imaging for other conditions. The prevalence of adrenal incidentalomas is approximately 2%, increasing with age to about 4% in middle-aged individuals and 10% in the elderly [24]. Importantly, ~90% of adrenocortical tumors are still >4 cm at diagnosis [24]. Thus, tumors larger than 4 cm or those that enlarge by 1 cm during the observation period typically warrant surgical removal following thorough endocrine evaluation [24].

Minimally invasive surgery, particularly PRLA, has significantly impacted the management of these tumors, improving patient outcomes without altering the fundamental indications and goals of treatment. However, it is important to recognize that PRLA may not be suitable for all patients or all adrenal pathologies [25]. Large tumors (>6–8 cm) or those with suspected malignancy may be better served by an open or transperitoneal approach, which allows for wider resection margins and minimizes the risk of tumor spillage [26]. Conversely, patients with extensive prior abdominal surgery or severe cardiopulmonary comorbidities may not be ideal candidates for anterior transperitoneal LA, due to intraperitoneal adhesions, which make it harder to tolerate transperitoneal insufflation pressure, as opposed to retroperitoneal [27].

The choice between laparoscopic and open adrenalectomy should be guided by a thorough evaluation of each case, considering factors such as tumor size, location, and the patient's overall health. A multidisciplinary approach, involving surgery, radiology, anesthesiology, and endocrinology, is essential to establish the best surgical strategy and ensure the best possible outcomes for patients. While LA has become the gold standard for most adrenal surgeries, open surgery remains a vital option for complex cases where minimally invasive techniques may not be feasible.

Despite the solid advantages of LA, there remain specific indications for open adrenalectomy. Open surgery is often preferred for malignant adrenal tumors, especially those >12 cm or involving neighboring structures, due to the fragility of such tumors and the risk of iatrogenic disease dissemination. Additionally, patients with significant cardiopulmonary issues, coagulopathy, or extensive previous abdominal or retroperitoneal surgeries may be better suited for open surgery. Conversion to open surgery during PRLA is a rare but necessary event, typically occurring in cases of clinically unforeseen intraoperative findings, such as the detection of more extensive local invasion or regional lymph node metastasis, or due to the inability to control intraoperative complications laparoscopically, i.e., aggressive bleeding due to surgical injuries to major vessels and/or inadvertent injury of surrounding organs [8]. The surgical team's experience, hospital volume, and a multidisciplinary approach to patient management are critical factors in minimizing the need for conversion and ensuring optimal outcomes.

Ultimately, the indications for PRLA, like other forms of LA, vary depending on the surgeon's expertise and the specific characteristics of the tumor. While larger tumors, malignant tumors, and pheochromocytomas present greater challenges, they are not absolute contraindications for PRLA. According to the Society of American Gastrointestinal and Endoscopic Surgeons (SAGES) guidelines, tumors $\geq$ 7.5 cm pose increased risks, including longer surgeries, more blood loss, extended hospital stays, and higher conversion rates to open surgery [10]. However, for small adrenocortical cancers and non-invasive metastatic adrenal tumors, the European Society for Medical Oncology (ESMO) guidelines recommend LA [28]. Studies have shown that outcomes for LA and open surgery in these cases are similar [28]. However, it is worth highlighting the importance of adhering to oncological safety surgical principles and converting to open surgery if necessary.

Contraindications to PRLA can be categorized into relative and absolute contraindications, centered around both patient factors and tumor characteristics. Patient body habitus plays a crucial role, with a body mass index (BMI) > 40 being generally considered a relative contraindication due to the limited working space in the retroperitoneum. Similarly, inadequate distance between the 12th rib and the posterior superior iliac crest can impede proper access and instrument maneuverability, potentially precluding the use of this approach. Tumor size and nature also factor into the decision-making process. Lesions larger than 7 cm pose challenges within the confined retroperitoneal space, while any suspicion of malignancy with potential invasion into surrounding structures may necessitate a more extensive surgical approach [25,29,30].

Absolute contraindications include the patient's inability to tolerate general anesthesia or maintain a prone position during the procedure, both of which are fundamental requirements for PRLA [1,31]. Confirmed invasion of the tumor into adjacent structures or extremely large tumors that cannot be safely manipulated within the retroperitoneal space also absolutely contraindicate this approach. It is important to note that these contraindications can sometimes be relative, depending on the surgeon's experience and specific patient circumstances. Some highly experienced surgeons might consider attempting PRLA in borderline cases, such as patients with a BMI slightly >40 or tumors marginally >7 cm, if other factors are favorable [18]. Additionally, while not an absolute contraindication, a history of extensive abdominal surgery may complicate the procedure due to potential adhesions and altered anatomy.

These contraindications underscore the importance of meticulous patient selection for PRLA to ensure optimal surgical outcomes and patient safety. As with any surgical technique, the decision to proceed with PRLA must be made on a case-by-case basis, carefully weighing the potential benefits against the risks and considering alternative approaches when necessary.

3. Comparative Morphology of the Adrenal Glands

The adrenal glands, also known as suprarenal glands—the targets of this surgical approach—are crucial endocrine organs with complex functions and an intricate, asymmetrical anatomy. Thus, these glands play a crucial role in secreting multiple distinct hormones, both cholesterol-/lipid- and protein-derived, essential for maintaining bodily homeostasis.

3.1. General Histological Structure

Herein, the adrenals consist of two histologically and functionally distinct tissue layers: the outer cortex (i.e., the superficial layer), and the central medulla (i.e., the inner deep layer), each wityh different embryological origins and producing different specialized hormones (see Figure 1).

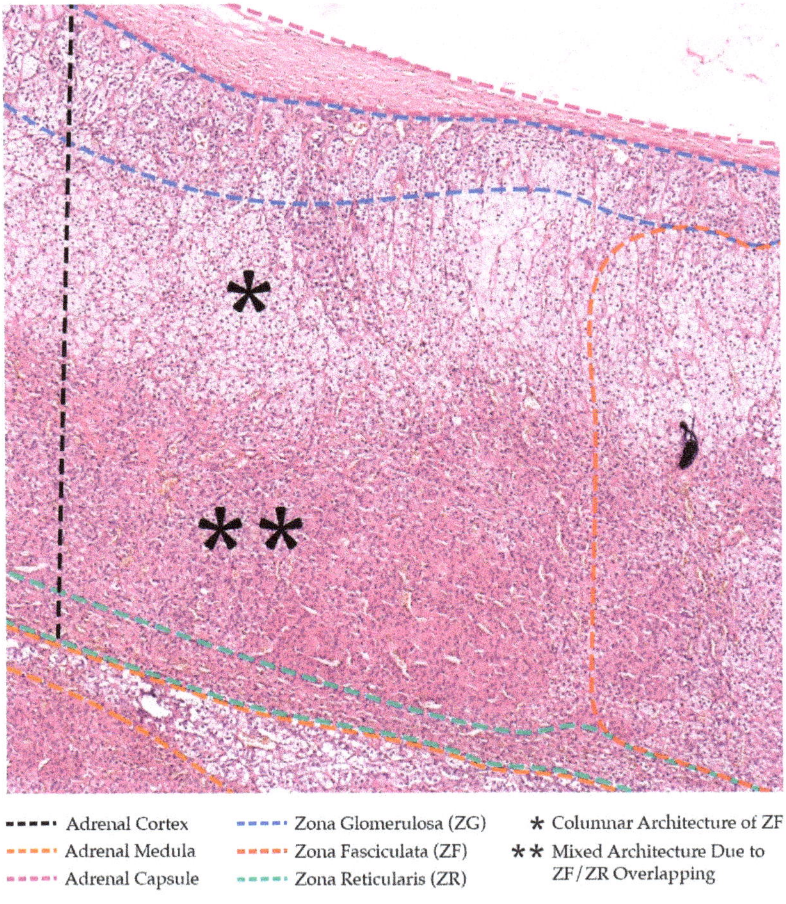

Figure 1. Histological architecture of the adrenal glands (hematoxylin–eosin, 100×).

The adrenal cortex is derived from mesenchymal cells attached to the coelomic cavity, adjacent to the urogenital ridge, proximal to the developing kidney, starting around the fourth week of intrauterine life. It secretes steroid hormones from three distinct zones of selectively specialized cortical tissue (see Figure 1), organized from external to internal: mineralocorticoids (e.g., aldosterone) in the zona glomerulosa (15–20% of the whole adrenal cortex), glucocorticoids (e.g., cortisol/cortisone) in the zona fasciculata (60–70%), and androgens (e.g., dehydroepiandrosterone—DHEA) in the zona reticularis (10–15%) [32].

These hormones regulate essential metabolic processes, such as the following: (1) aldosterone—hydroelectrolytic balance and blood pressure regulation; (2) cortisol—glucose metabolism homeostasis, through gluconeogenesis following proteic and lipidic lysis, and immune response modulation, through inflammation suppression; (3) DHEA—precursor androgen for the synthesis of other steroids (estrogen, progesterone, testosterone, and cortisol), which will be converted to fully functional sex hormones in the gonads or other target organs, playing a role in the development of secondary sexual traits and, thus, mitigating sexual function [32,33].

Conversely, the adrenal medulla, originating from ectodermal neural crest cells, represents an integral part of the sympathetic nervous system (i.e., considered to be a specialized sympathetic ganglion, yet lacking distinct synapses and releasing its secretion directly into the bloodstream). These ectodermal neural crest cells migrate to the cortex in the seventh week of gestation and gradually invade it, differentiating into chromaffin cells in response to cortisol, and ultimately forming the medulla centrally, supplied by plexus arteries and capillaries penetrating the cortex and constituting the cortico-medullary portal system. Thus, although lacking a clear histological border with the cortex, the adrenal medulla accounts for ~10% of the total adrenal gland volume (see Figure 1) [33].

Further migration of these adreno-medullary cells—called chromaffin cells due to their brown-staining cytoplasmic granules, seen with chromium salts—as (nor)epinephrine oxidizes to melanin, explains the existence of ectopic adrenal tissues, often located near the aorta and vertebral column, i.e., paraganglia—chromaffin cell clusters distributed on both sides of the aorta. The organ of Zuckerkandl, positioned near the inferior mesenteric artery, represents the largest accumulation of chromaffin cells outside the adrenal medulla. This organ serves as the primary source of catecholamines during the first year of life [34].

Preganglionic sympathetic neurons, which regulate the adrenal medulla, receive synaptic inputs from neurons in the pons, medulla, and hypothalamus. This neuronal connection allows the brain to control sympathetic activity. The medulla responds to sympathetic preganglionic neuron stimulation (i.e., thoracic preganglionic fibers originating at the level of T5-T11) by secreting tyrosine-derived catecholamines (e.g., epinephrine and norepinephrine, dopamine), which are neurotransmitters that are critical for rapid stress responses (i.e., the body's fight-or-flight response) [33].

3.2. Bilateral Gross Anatomy

Macroscopically, these suprarenal glands have a golden yellow–grayish appearance, due to the high contents of intracellular lipids within the cortex, and a firm consistency. Encased posterolaterally by the 10th–12th ribs on the left, and by the 11th–12th ribs on the right, the surprarenals typically weigh 4–8 g, measuring 4–5 cm in length and 2–4 cm in width, in adults. In contrast, they are proportionally larger in newborns, constituting approximately 20–25% of the total body weight [32].

Anatomically, these small (yet vital), triangular-shaped, paired endocrine glands are located deep in the supero-posterior abdomen (projected anteriorly at the level of the epigastrium), nestled within the uppermost part of the retroperitoneum, immediately above the kidneys. Their name, derived from the Latin "ad renalis", meaning "near the kidney", aptly describes their location, namely, superiorly and antero-medially along the upper poles of the kidneys, within the paravertebral gutters, flanking the vertebral column at the level of T12 (T11-L1) bilaterally [34]. However, the precise shape and location of each adrenal gland differ slightly from one side to the other. This asymmetry in location and shape is an important consideration for surgeons as they plan and execute their approach.

Thus, as does the right kidney compared to the left, the right adrenal lies lower and more medial to the spine than the left adrenal. Moreover, the right adrenal gland is also thicker and taller, with a more pyramidal shape, being positioned posterior to the inferior vena cava (IVC), within the angle between the right lobe of the liver and the right crus of the diaphragm, with its anterior surface abutting the posterolateral surface of the retro-hepatic IVC, separated by only a thin layer of fascial connective tissue [1,32]. Thus, the IVC isolates the anterior surface of the right adrenal from the more anterior Winslow foramen, the second duodenal segment, and the cephalic pancreas. Lying anterior to the diaphragm and lateral to the right diaphragmatic crus, it is usually covered antero-superiorly and supero-laterally by the "bare area" of the liver or the right hepatic lobe, respectively [35], whereas infero-laterally, the anterior surface may at times be covered by the peritoneum, the liver, and hepatic flexure of the colon [36]. The anterior aspect of the right adrenal may also, albeit rarely, come into contact with the first segment of the duodenum inferiorly. The posterior surface of the right adrenal is divided by a ridge, nestled against the diaphragm superiorly, and against the supero-medial upper pole of the ipsilateral kidney inferiorly. Due to its high suprarenal position, the right adrenal characteristically does not reach the ipsilateral renal hilum, lacking proximity to the right renal vessels [1].

Comparatively, the left adrenal is larger, with a more flattened, semilunar/crescent shape, and lies more antero-medial than superior in relation to the ipsilateral kidney, as compared to the right side [32]. Contrastingly, as it lies partially in front of the left kidney, the left adrenal plunges anteriorly towards the renal hilum, being in close proximity to the left renal vessels with its inferior aspect. Furthermore, the left adrenal is situated posterolateral to the abdominal aorta (~7 mm away), anterior to the diaphragm, with its posterior surface in contact with the left diaphragmatic crus, yet posterior to the stomach, spleen/splenic vessels, and pancreas, and superior—albeit antero-medially—to the upper pole of the left kidney [37]. Superiorly, its anterior surface is closely related to the posterior peritoneal wall of the omental bursa (lesser sac), which, in turn, separates the gland from both the spleen and the cardia of the stomach [32,37]. The inferior portion of the anterior surface, however, lacks peritoneal coverage. Instead, it is in direct contact with the body and tail of the pancreas, as well as the splenic blood vessels [37].

Perirenal fatty tissue surrounds the adrenals bilaterally, both being enclosed within the ipsilateral perirenal fascia, with the exception of the connective tissue segment separating them from the kidneys [32]. This shared fascial envelope is a key anatomical feature that surgeons exploit during PRLA, as the perirenal compartment helps define the surgical plane of dissection. Positioned immediately beneath the diaphragm, the adrenal glands are anchored to the diaphragmatic crura via the renal fascia. Fibrous tissue bands attach the adrenals to the abdominal wall/diaphragm [32]. Thus, it is worth noting that the aforementioned connective tissue segment that separates the adrenal gland from the kidney also becomes important during the dissection phase of the surgery.

These complex anatomical relationships underscore the importance of a thorough understanding of regional anatomy when performing PRLA. The surgeon must navigate carefully around these structures to safely access and remove the adrenal gland.

3.3. *Vascularization, Lymphatics and Innervation*

The vascular supply of the adrenal glands is as complex and asymmetrical as their location. Among the most highly perfused organs, the adrenal glands receive 2000 mL/kg/min of the circulating blood volume, ranking third in perfusion after the thyroid and kidneys [38]. Thus, the adrenal glands receive this rich blood supply from three main homologous arteries on each side, forming a dense arterial subcapsular plexus around the gland. As shown in Figure 2, these are as follows:

1. The superior adrenal arteries: Usually one to three, but up to six to eight per side, the superior adrenal arterial branches arise from the inferior phrenic arteries, before they distribute to the diaphragm, and supply the upper part of the glands.
2. The middle adrenal arteries: Though inconsistent—i.e., single, multiple, or absent—they supply the perirenal fat only, emerging directly from the abdominal aorta, just proximal to the origin of the renal artery. Reaching the inner side of the adrenal, the middle

adrenal artery gives branches on both glandular surfaces. On the right side, these branches cross the IVC in a retro-caval manner.

3. The inferior adrenal arteries: One, or at times multiple, these inferior braches arise from the main renal artery, or an accessory or superior polar renal artery, with small collaterals even originating in the superior ureteric artery, and enter the gland through its inferior surface [32–34].

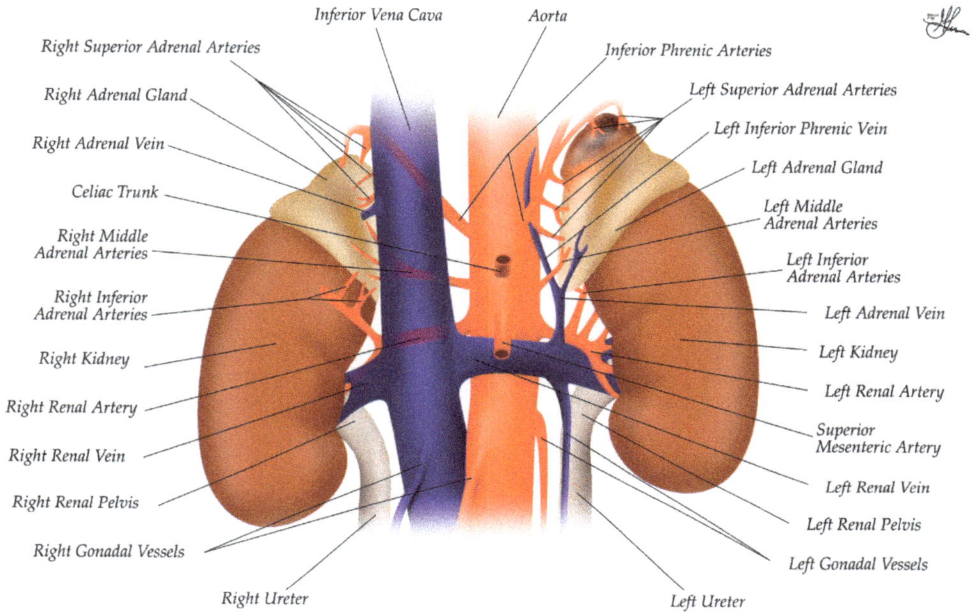

Figure 2. Illustration of bilateral adrenal gland vascularization: anterior view, coronal section.

In addition to these main sources, the adrenal glands may also receive blood supply from small arteries originating from the subcostal and gonadal vessels. Herein, the main branches divide before entering the glandular tissue and ramify [32]. There may be up to 50 arterioles creating an intricate network under the adrenal capsule, i.e., the subcapsular arterial plexus [1]. Thereafter, sinusoids draw their origin and descend inward, around clusters of glomerulosa cells, in between the zona fasciculata columns, to form a deep capillary plexus in the innermost zona reticularis of the adrenal cortex (see Figure 1). This plexus will provide drainage to the medullary veins [1]. This abundant vascularity is a double-edged sword for surgeons—while it ensures the vitality of the gland, it also increases the risk of troublesome bleeding during surgery if vessels are inadvertently injured.

Venous drainage of the adrenal glands is also asymmetrical and is not correspondent to the arterial system. At the level of the gland's hilum, a singular consolidated adrenal vein emerges, draining the entire gland. Herein, as the left adrenal vein emerges from the hilum and descends along the anterior surface of the left adrenal gland, it is joined by the left inferior phrenic vein, before ultimately emptying into the left renal vein (see Figure 2). This arrangement creates a longer path for venous drainage on the left side. In contrast, the right adrenal vein follows a more direct route. After emerging from the hilum, it courses obliquely and drains directly into the posterior aspect of the IVC (see Figure 2). This shorter, more direct path can present unique challenges during surgical procedures [32–34,39].

In summary, the right suprarenal vein is typically short (~5 mm in length) and drains directly into the IVC on its posterolateral aspect, whereas the left suprarenal vein is longer (~3 cm) and drains into the left renal vein or occasionally into the inferior phrenic vein (see Figure 2) [24]. Adding to this complexity, variations in venous anatomy—particularly on the right side, where the short adrenal vein can be challenging to dissect and control—can affect the surgical approach and technique.

In fact, anatomical variations in adrenal venous drainage are not uncommon (in ~12.8% of patients), especially on the right side. The right adrenal vein may drain into a posterior hepatic vein (1.6% of cases), into the IVC just below a hepatic vein (6.3% of cases), or there may be two adrenal veins draining into the IVC (3.1% of cases). When an adrenal shows two distinct venous trunks at the level of the hilum, they are usually disposed as follows: one main trunk, following the conventional aforementioned course, and on accessory trunks, which drain into the inferior phrenic vein. Occasionally, the right adrenal vein may drain into the IVC immediately above the renal vein [39]. These variations underscore the need for careful preoperative imaging and intraoperative vigilance.

The lymphatic drainage of the adrenal glands is also worth noting. Two lymphatic plexuses exist within each gland—one beneath the capsule and another inside the medulla. These plexuses channel lymph into several node groups: renal hilum nodes, para-aortic nodes (specifically those proximal to the diaphragmatic crux/renal artery), and para-caval nodes. Some lymphatic vessels even traverse the diaphragm via the minute orifices housing splanchnic nerves, thus draining towards the thoracic duct, as well as the pre-vertebral/dorsal mediastinal lymph nodes [40]. This complex lymphatic drainage system explains the pattern of distant dissemination sometimes seen in adrenal cancer [32].

Relative to their size, the adrenal glands have the largest autonomic supply out of all human organs. Their innervation is derived from multiple sources: the celiac and renal plexuses, and the thoracic splanchnic nerves. These nerve fibers form the suprarenal plexus, which can be further divided into three secondary plexuses: the adreno-celiac, adreno-renal, and adreno-diaphragmatic plexuses. This rich innervation disposes itself between the inner aspect of each gland and the medial celiac/aorto-renal ganglia. It consists mainly of preganglionic sympathetic fibers, which permeate deep within the gland, to finally synapse with the medullary chromaffin cells [40]. This conformation is essential for the rapid secretion of catecholamines in response to stress. Albeit in smaller proportion, post-ganglionic sympathetic fibers also exist, to innervate the cortical blood vessels [32–34].

3.4. Surgical Implications for PRLA

Vascular control is a critical step in PRLA. Early ligation of the adrenal vein is important to prevent the release of catecholamines. From a posterior perspective, the right adrenal gland presents unique anatomical considerations. The right adrenal vein, a critical structure for ligation during adrenalectomy, is situated posterior to the gland, between it and the IVC. This positioning requires meticulous dissection/mobilization of the right suprarenal gland to ensure proper identification/ligation of the vein. Conversely, the left suprarenal gland offers a somewhat more straightforward approach. The left adrenal vein is typically identified at the infero-medial border of the gland, generally allowing for easier dissection and ligation compared to its right-sided counterpart. However, the left adrenal's position relative to the kidney introduces its own complexities [41].

Exposure of the adrenal gland requires the mobilization of perirenal fat, identification of the upper pole of the kidney as an initial landmark, and medial/caudal retraction of the kidney to expose the adrenal gland. The left adrenal gland falls in front of the upper pole antero-medially, descending towards the renal hilum, and thus necessitates more extensive mobilization of the left kidney as compared to the right. This anatomical arrangement has significant implications for surgical technique and approach [32,41].

Complete mobilization of the adrenal gland requires attention to its anatomical attachments. Medially, it must be dissected from the diaphragmatic crus. Laterally, it is separated from the kidney. Superiorly, attachments to the diaphragm must be divided. Anteriorly, careful separation from surrounding structures such as the liver or pancreas is necessary. The plane between the adrenal gland and the kidney is typically avascular, allowing for preservation of the renal vasculature [31].

Several anatomical factors can present challenges during PRLA. Obesity can obscure landmarks and limit the working space due to excess retroperitoneal fat. Previous retroperitoneal surgery may result in altered anatomy and scarring. Large tumors can distort the normal anatomy and further restrict the already limited working space. Right-sided tumors present a particular challenge due to their proximity to the IVC, increasing the risk of vascular injury. Pheochromocytomas, with their increased vascularity and friable tissue, require extra caution [1,3].

Common anatomical pitfalls to avoid during PRLA include injury to the diaphragm or pleura during superior dissection, inadvertent entry into the peritoneal cavity, injury to renal vessels during adrenal dissection, avulsion of the short right adrenal vein, and injury to surrounding organs such as the liver, pancreas, or spleen [3].

Understanding the detailed anatomy of the adrenal glands and their surrounding structures is essential for effective and safe surgical interventions, particularly in procedures like PRLA. Mastery of these anatomical nuances enhances surgical precision and patient outcomes. The adrenal glands are vital endocrine organs that play a significant role in the body's hormonal regulation. Their intricate vascular, lymphatic, and neural networks, coupled with their distinct anatomical positions and relationships with adjacent structures, require thorough knowledge and precision in surgical practices. The transition to a posterior anatomical view in PRLA represents a significant shift from traditional approaches, emphasizing the need for a comprehensive understanding of the adrenal glands' anatomy to ensure successful outcomes in adrenal surgery.

4. Relevant Surgical Topography and Anatomical Landmarks for PRLA

PRLA constitutes a unique approach to adrenal gland removal that challenges traditional surgical perspectives. At its core, PRLA represents a so-called "backdoor" approach [18], which quite literally rotates the conventional adrenal surgery overview 180 degrees. Unlike the more familiar transperitoneal laparoscopic technique, the fundamental premise of PRLA involves positioning the patient prone, with trocar access incisions being made posteriorly, bypassing the peritoneal cavity entirely and facilitating direct access to the adrenals. However, this seemingly simple change in orientation brings with it a plethora of anatomical considerations that surgeons must grapple with. Thus, while the adrenal anatomy remains consistent regardless of approach, surgeons must adapt to a more confined working space and shift their mental model to a posterior anatomical view—a perspective that diverges significantly from traditional surgical training. Despite its advantages, the unfamiliarity of surgeons with the posterior anatomical perspective has thus far been the main limiting factor regarding the widespread adoption of PRLA [15].

Even so, PRLA offers significant benefits over traditional approaches, provided the surgeon has a thorough understanding of the complex anatomy of the adrenal glands and retroperitoneal space. The reduced operative time, less postoperative pain, and minimized risk of intra-abdominal complications make PRLA an attractive option. However, the limited working space and the need for anatomical orientation pose challenges. Surgeons must adapt to the posterior perspective, which can be challenging without sufficient anatomical familiarity. This section discusses critical retroperitoneal topography and abdominal parietal architecture, emphasizing their practical implications for PRLA.

4.1. Parietal Anatomy for Trocar Placement

The anatomical positioning of the adrenal gland determines the placement of trocars in the "backdoor" approach. Thus, the efficacy of PRLA is contingent upon precise trocar placement, which necessitates a comprehensive understanding of the abdominal wall's layered anatomy. The abdominal cavity is bordered by three anatomically distinct walls: superior (the diaphragm), posterior, and antero-lateral.

The antero-lateral abdominal wall comprises the rectus abdominis, the pyramidalis, the transversus abdominis (TA), the internal oblique (IO), and the external oblique (EO) muscles. During PRLA, surgical access only involves the posterior half of the antero-lateral abdominal wall. As depicted in Figure 3, this posterior half area includes three large muscles (from superficial to deep): the EO, IO, and TA muscles, separated individually by thin layers of connective tissue. The transversalis fascia nearly completely covers the deep surface of the TA muscle. Anteriorly, these three muscles terminate through a common aponeurosis, which distributes itself to encase the rectus muscle and form the linea alba anteriorly, at the midline [42].

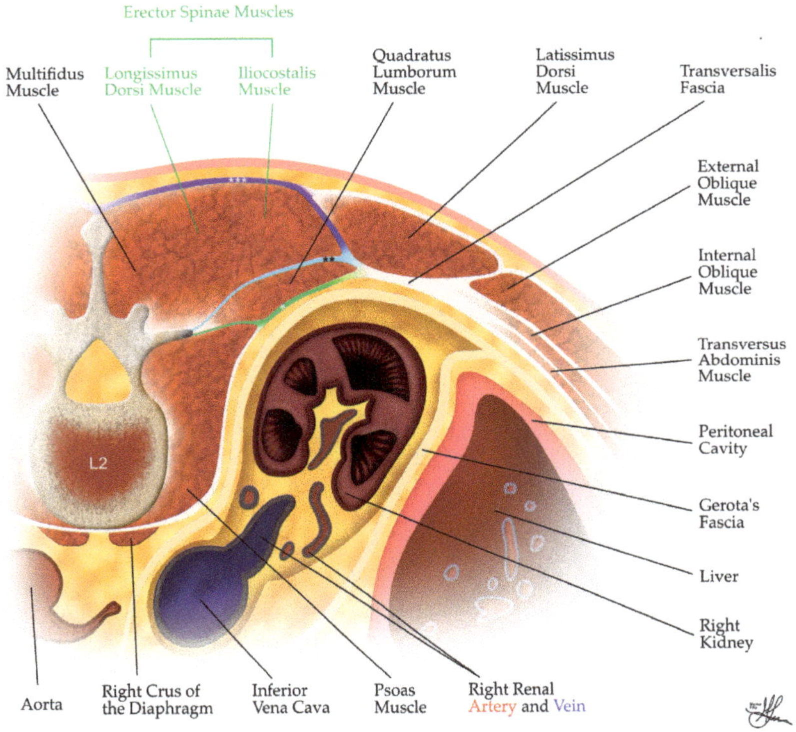

Figure 3. Abdominal parietal anatomy illustration, focusing on the right posterior and antero-lateral walls, in an axial L2 section of a prone patient, superior view. *—Anterior layer of thoracolumbar fascia (marked in green); **—middle layer of thoracolumbar fascia (marked in light blue); ***—posterior layer of thoracolumbar fascia (marked in deep blue).

The anatomy of the posterior abdominal wall is another crucial consideration in PRLA. Herein, this posterior wall includes the spine and two lumbo-iliac regions, symmetric bilaterally, bordered cranially by the 12th rib, laterally by the lateral border of the quadratus lumborum, caudally by the iliac crest, and medially by the spine (see Figure 4). This area contains three groups of muscles and serves as the medial landmark for performing PRLA. These muscle groups are described, from dorsal to ventral, as follows:

1. The dorsal group comprises the latissimus dorsi muscle and its aponeurosis (see Figure 3), the serratus posterior inferior muscle (see Figure 4), and the erector spinae (ES) muscle group, i.e., comprising the longissimus dorsi and iliocostalis muscles in the lumbar region (see Figure 3).
2. The middle group consists of the dorsal insertion of the TA muscle aponeurosis and the intertransverse process muscles (i.e., intertransversarii, transversospinales/multifidus muscle—see Figure 3).
3. The ventral group, located ventral to the TA aponeurosis, includes the quadratus lumborum and the psoas muscles (see Figure 3) [32,42].

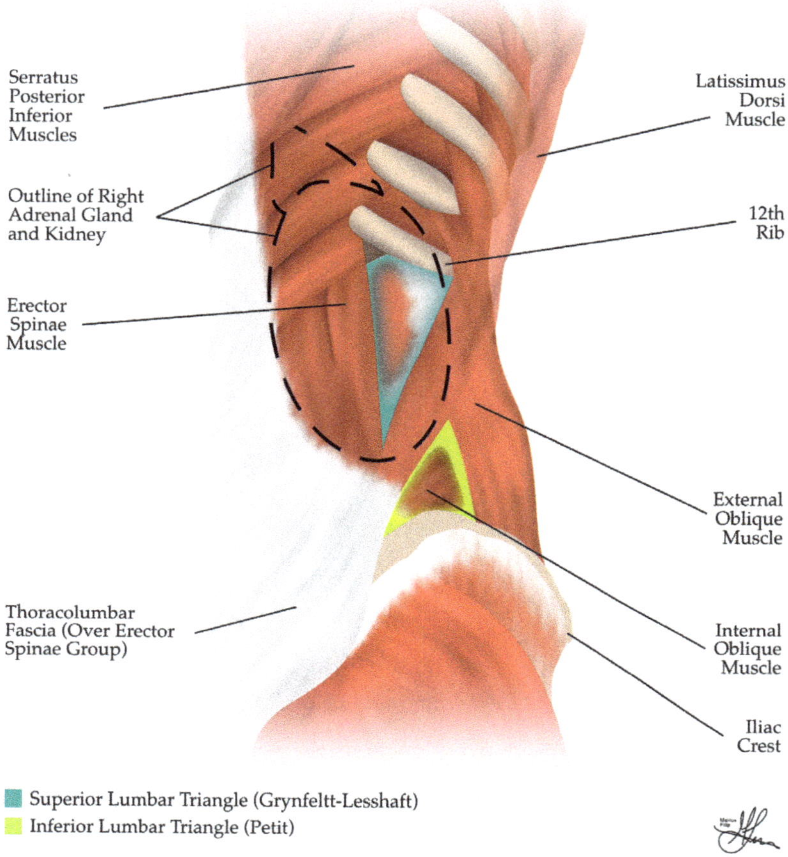

Figure 4. Posterior abdominal wall anatomy illustration: right side, posterior view, coronal section.

During PRLA, trocar placement occurs lateral to the lumbo-iliac region, with the lateral border of the ES muscle group, in particular, serving as the central medial landmark for trocar positioning (see Figure 4). The fasciae of the posterior abdominal wall are equally important. The thoracolumbar fascia, a thin fibrous layer, covers most of the aforementioned muscles (see Figure 4) and is divided into three sagittal layers: the anterior layer (marked *, in green, in Figure 3), which covers the quadratus lumborum, alongside the middle (marked **, in light blue, in Figure 3) and posterior (marked ***, in deep blue, in Figure 3) layers, which envelop the ES muscles and unite towards the lateral border of the ES group to form a strong raphe. Thereafter, the raphe is reached by the aforementioned anterior layer, forming the aponeurosis of the TA muscle at the lateral border of the quadratus lumborum [42] (see Figure 3). The transversalis fascia, which lines the deep surface of the TA muscle, and the psoas fascia, covering the psoas muscle, are also important anatomical features to be aware of (see Figure 3).

The Grynfeltt–Lesshaft triangle, or superior lumbar triangle (see Figure 4), is typically penetrated by the medial trocar during PRLA. This triangle is bounded laterally by the dorsal border of the IO muscle, medially by the lateral border of the ES muscles, and cranially by the 12th rib. Occasionally, the triangle assumes a square shape, when the angle between the 12th rib and the spinal muscles is covered by the serratus posterior inferior muscle. Within this triangle, the TA aponeurosis is directly covered by the latissimus dorsi muscle [32,43]. The Grynfeltt triangle is a weak point of the abdominal wall and is prone to herniation. The true weak point is the lateral half, where the TA aponeurosis is perforated by vessels and nerves, as the medial half is ventrally covered by the quadratus lumborum [44,45] (see Figure 3).

The Petit triangle, or inferior lumbar triangle (see Figure 4), is another area of weakness and potential herniation, observed when the latissimus dorsi muscle does not extend to the EO muscle. The boundaries of this triangle are the dorsal edge of the EO muscle laterally, the lateral free edge of the latissimus dorsi medially, and the posterior superior iliac crest bone inferiorly [43]. The Petit triangle, located inferior to the operative field, is generally not accessed during PRLA but may be inadvertently punctured when mounting an additional fourth trocar, if deemed necessary for retraction and achieving adequate exposure [31].

The blood supply to the posterior abdominal wall comes from the posterior ramifications of the intercostal arteries, lumbar arteries (arising from the posterior aspect of the abdominal aorta), and lateral sacral arteries (arising from the posterior divisions of the internal iliac arteries) [32]. Conversely, for the antero-lateral wall, perfusion is provided mainly by the superior and inferior epigastric and the deep circumflex iliac arteries, with some minor branches of the intercostal and lumbar vessels also present [42]. Venous drainage mirrors the arterial architecture. Generally, there is no risk of damaging these vascular structures during PRLA. However, awareness of their presence and course is important for honing one's comprehensive anatomical understanding.

In contrast, the innervation of the posterior abdominal wall deserves special attention due to the risk of inadvertent injury during PRLA. The skin covering the back receives sensitive innervation from the spinal nerves, through their posterior rami. Thus, posterior cutaneous incisions, especially those more proximal to the midline, may be associated with temporary peri-incisional numbness, which is generally self-limiting and typically resolves on its own over time, as it would in any other area of the body [32].

Furthermore, the intercostal nerves, constituting the anterior rami of the spinal nerves, course along the caudal margins of the ribs, beneath the intercostal arteries. These mixed nerves provide somatic muscular branches to the intercostal muscles, as well as sensitive cutaneous branches (lateral and anterior) for the skin of the antero-lateral abdominal wall. Herein, ventral to the mid-axillary line, these lateral cutaneous branches of the intercostal nerves pierce the intercostal muscles and emerge through the parietal muscles to give sensitive cutaneous innervation [32].

Due to this anatomical conformation, the T12 intercostal nerve is actually subcostal, running along the caudal margin of the 12th rib and, thus, being particularly vulnerable during central and medial port placement. Initially, the subcostal T12 nerve emerges anterior to the quadratus lumborum and then travels between the TA and the IO muscles [42], only to subsequently follow the same distribution pattern as its counterparts, i.e., the other intercostal nerves. The lateral cutaneous branch of the T12 subcostal nerve emerges near the lateral edge of the quadratus lumborum, perforates the posterior parietal abdominal muscles, and becomes subcutaneous at the midpoint of the iliac crest, giving rise to several branches responsible for the cutaneous sensory innervation of the hip and gluteal regions [32]. Other relevant nerves include the iliohypogastric and ilioinguinal nerves (both L1), which run parallel and inferior to the subcostal nerve, and the lateral cutaneous nerve of the thigh (L2-3), which crosses the iliac crest. Caution is advised regarding horizontal incisions and large sutures, as these can entrap/transect nerves supplying motor innervation, increasing the risk of hernias/pseudo-hernias [32,42].

In summary, several surface anatomical landmarks are crucial for successful PRLA. The 12th rib serves as the superior limit of retroperitoneal access, while the posterior superior iliac crest defines the inferior limit. The ES muscles constitute the medial limit for port placement, and the posterior axillary line marks the lateral limit. It is worth noting that the adrenal glands themselves are encased by the 10th–12th ribs, providing some natural protection but also potentially limiting access. When accessing the retroperitoneum below the 12th rib, caution is advised in order to avoid injury to the T12 intercostal nerve, thus preventing abdominal wall relaxation or hypoesthesia. Ideally, during PRLA, the muscles of the abdominal wall that are traversed by the trocars should only include the latissimus dorsi, EO, IO, and TA. The paravertebral muscles, such as the ES and quadratus lumborum, should typically not be affected during the procedure, as they define the limit for medial trocar placement.

4.2. Retroperitoneal Topography

Understanding the anatomy of the retroperitoneal cavity is crucial for successful PRLA. For a proper management of the spatial relationships encountered during PRLA, this approach necessitates a thorough understanding of the retroperitoneum's tripartite division into the following compartments:

1. The anterior pararenal space (marked 1, in green, in Figure 5), bordered anteriorly by the posterior parietal peritoneum (****) and posteriorly by the anterior perirenal fascia (Gerota's fascia *). While not directly accessed during PRLA, it contains multiple vital structures: the ascending (right side) or descending (left side) colon laterally, and the duodenum, pancreas, and the mesenteric root of the small bowel centrally and medially. Although this posterior approach minimizes the risk of injury to these structures, their proximity underscores the importance of maintaining anatomical orientation throughout the procedure.
2. The perirenal space (marked 2, in pink, in Figure 5), bound within the perirenal fascia, contains the kidneys, adrenals, and proximal ureters, surrounded by perirenal fat. It is accessed by incising the perirenal fascia and represents the main workspace for PRLA.
3. The posterior pararenal space (marked 3, in blue, in Figure 5), delimitated between the posterior perirenal fascia (Zuckerkandl's fascia **) anteriorly and the posterior abdominal wall musculature (quadratus lumborum, TA, and the thoracolumbar fascia) posteriorly. It is devoid of major organs and represents the first compartment accessed by the surgeon during PRLA, being then traversed sagittally to reach the more anterior perirenal workspace [32,46].

The retroperitoneal spaces are separated by avascular interfascial planes, a fact that surgeons can leverage to minimize bleeding during dissection. Moreover, these spaces extend through the posterior midline, adjoin the liver's bare area and the hemidiaphragms bilaterally, and converge in the pelvis. This anatomical continuity creates potential routes for fluid or pathological dissemination between the thoracic and pelvic regions, a factor that must be considered in both surgical planning and postoperative care [47].

The fascial layers of the retroperitoneum play a crucial role in PRLA (see Figure 5). Gerota's fascia (*), also known as the perirenal fascia, envelops both the kidney and the adrenal gland, forming the perirenal space. This fascia is divided into anterior (*) and posterior layers (**). The lateroconal fascia (***) extends from the transversalis fascia laterally [46]. These fascial planes are key to defining the surgical approach and guiding dissection during PRLA. The posterior approach used in PRLA enters the retroperitoneum behind Gerota's fascia, providing a direct route to the adrenal gland.

Conversely, the surgical approach in PRLA leverages this anatomical arrangement to great effect. The procedure initiates with an incision through the abdominal wall, specifically lateral to the lumbo-iliac area. This entry point is strategically chosen to optimize access while minimizing the risk of iatrogenic injury. From this initial incision, the surgeon navigates through the posterior pararenal space before directly accessing the perirenal space through the perirenal fascia. A key advantage of this approach lies in the relative absence of vital structures within the posterior pararenal space. This anatomical "safe zone" significantly mitigates the risk of inadvertent visceral injury during the initial phases of the procedure. This feature is particularly advantageous when compared to traditional transperitoneal approaches, where the risk of injury to intra-abdominal organs is inherently higher [41].

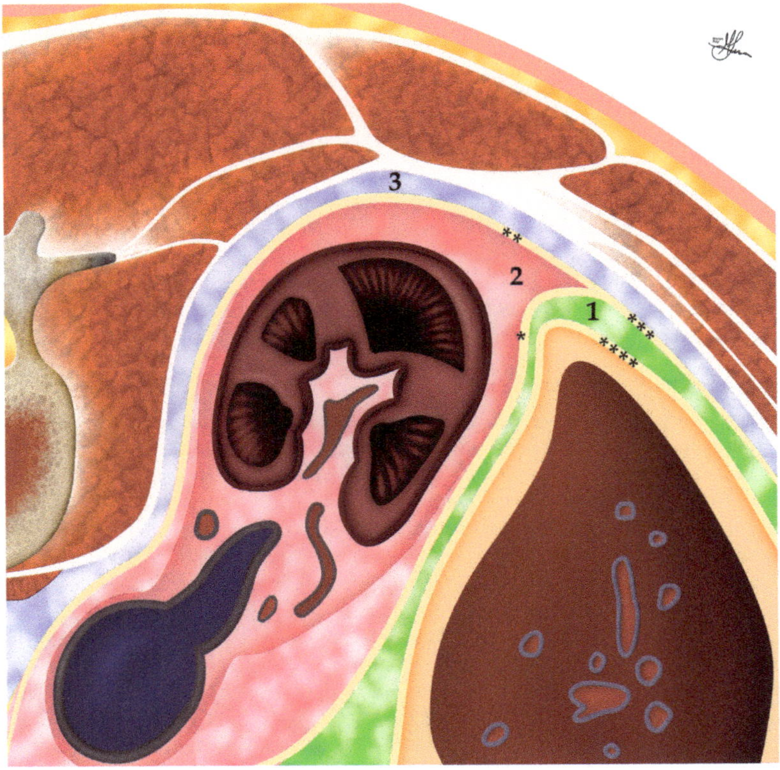

Figure 5. Illustration of the right retroperitoneal cavity, with highlighted fascial layers and compartmentation into retroperitoneal spaces: 1—anterior pararenal space (in green); 2—perirenal space (in pink); 3—posterior pararenal space (in blue); *—anterior perirenal fascia (Gerota's fascia); **—posterior perirenal fascia (Zuckerkandl's fascia); ***—lateroconal fascia; ****—posterior parietal peritoneum.

The "backdoor" nature of PRLA thus represents not merely a change in surgical perspective but a fundamental shift in how surgeons interact with the retroperitoneal anatomy. By exploiting the natural avascular planes and relatively safe, yet confined, spaces of the retroperitoneum, PRLA offers a pathway to the adrenal glands that minimizes disruption to surrounding structures while maintaining a clear and direct route to the surgical target, constituting a promising technique for adrenal surgery, which balances direct access with minimized risk [1]. However, its successful implementation is contingent upon a comprehensive understanding of the retroperitoneal anatomy from a posterior perspective. This includes not only the spatial relationships of the adrenal glands and surrounding structures, but also the broader anatomical context of the retroperitoneal spaces.

The unique viewpoint required for PRLA challenges traditional surgical perspectives, necessitating a mental reorientation from anterior to posterior anatomical conceptualization. As surgical education and training evolve to incorporate this approach, PRLA may become increasingly prevalent in clinical practice. Further research into the long-term outcomes and potential applications of this technique will be crucial in defining its role in the surgical management of adrenal pathologies.

5. Achieving Adequate Surgical Exposure

To perform PRLA, standard laparoscopic equipment and instruments are required. This technique can be executed by any surgical department. Even so, standardizing the steps of the PRLA procedure is essential during the initial learning phase. This standardized approach is particularly useful at the beginning of the learning curve. However, dynamic procedural modifications may become necessary, depending on intraoperative findings. A skilled and experienced surgeon must be adaptable to varying situations. Experience gained from various minimally invasive procedures is invaluable, as techniques learned in one procedure can often be applied to another. Surgeons with prior laparoscopic experience can generally reduce the learning curve for PRLA significantly.

Achieving an adequate surgical exposure of the adrenals, within a well-defined, clean operative field, constitutes the main initial hurdle for clinicians beginning to implement this approach. In this section, we explore the factors involved in achieving this overarching operative goal, i.e., the positioning of the patient and surgical team, the technical aspects of trocar placement, and the principles involved in developing an adequate retroperitoneal workspace laparoscopically.

5.1. Surgical Team and Patient Positioning

The prone jackknife position, commonly used in PRLA, presents specific challenges. Although it generally does not pose significant issues for mechanical ventilation, it can increase the risk of complications such as accidental extubation, nerve injuries, and cardiovascular events (especially in the context of IVC manipulation). Anesthesia teams must be prepared for these complications and should be trained to manage emergencies in the prone position, including accidental extubation or cardiac arrest [48]. Positioning-related injuries, such as pressure-induced nerve damage or ophthalmic complications, must be meticulously prevented through careful positioning and regular monitoring. The risk of venous gas embolism, while low, should also be considered, particularly during CO_2 insufflation [49].

Patients generally receive a prophylactic dose of preoperative antibiotics. A central venous catheter and an arterial line are usually required, especially for right-sided adrenalectomies, pheochromocytomas, or in the context of preexisting cardiovascular risks. In the supine position, sequential compression devices are applied for deep venous thrombosis prophylaxis, and general anesthesia induction and endotracheal intubation are achieved [50]. Thereafter, as seen in Figure 6, the patient is repositioned into a prone jackknife position. To achieve this, the surgical table must allow for adjustments to be made, to achieve an almost 90° hip flexion and to support bent knees, while ideally also allowing the abdomen to hang freely (Cloward Prone Positioner), reducing pressure on the retroperitoneal space [41]. Herein, it is important to position the superior anterior iliac crests correctly so that the abdominal wall is free and not restricted by hip supports, as the thighs are positioned with supported knees. Alternatively, a roll can be placed under the anterior iliac crests and another under the patient's thorax, facilitating the movement of the abdominal viscera away from the retroperitoneum, which is vital for creating an adequate working space [15]. Adjustable supports attached to the operating table should be used to align with the patient's body size.

The anesthesia team pads the patient's face and uses a mirror on the table to monitor the endotracheal tube's position. The table is set with little to no Trendelenburg tilt. The patient's arms are flexed and pronated on arm boards, with elbows bent at 90°, and the hips and knees are also bent at 90°, with all pressure points adequately padded. The knee rest is lowered to reduce pressure on the knees and prevent posterior displacement of the hips, which could interfere with instrument manipulation. Attention to detail in this setup phase is crucial, as it facilitates the surgical procedure [15,41].

Overall, the jackknife position may prove beneficial for increasing the distance between trocars, facilitating the manipulation of instruments within the limited working space. Thus, with the hips flexed at a 90° angle to maximize the space between the 12th rib and the iliac crest, this position provides optimal exposure for port placement and surgical access in PRLA. Moreover, this position has several further favorable anatomical implications. The position causes the abdominal contents to fall anteriorly, creating more working space in the retroperitoneum. It also shifts the kidneys caudally, improving exposure of the adrenal glands, and moves the diaphragm cranially, potentially improving respiratory mechanics. Finally, the posterior abdominal wall is stretched in this position, facilitating port placement [41].

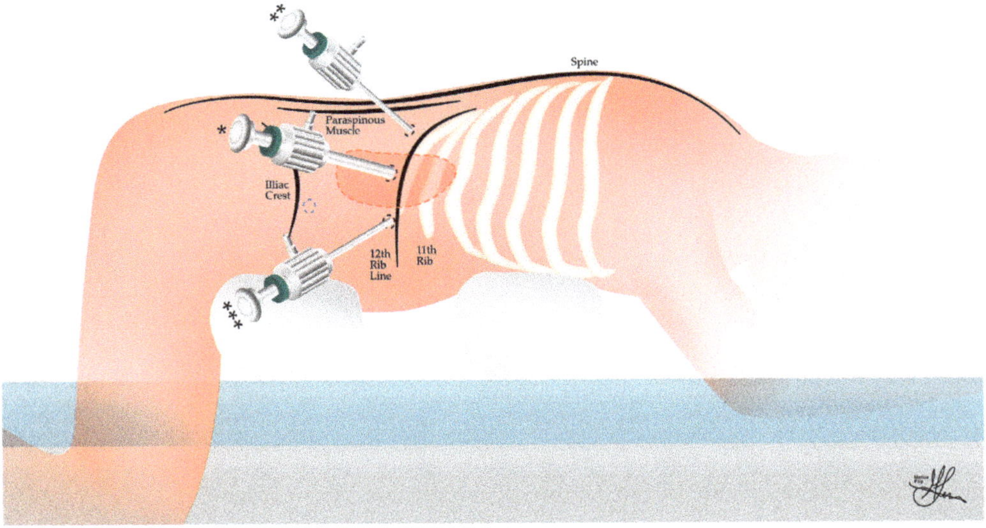

Figure 6. Prone jackknife positioning for posterior retroperitoneal laparoscopic adrenalectomy. *—Central 10 mm trocar; **—medial 5 mm trocar; ***—lateral 5 mm trocar; blue circle—optional additional 5 mm trocar, at times necessary for retraction.

The surgical team consists of the surgeon, the scopist, and the scrub nurse. The surgeon and the scopist are positioned on the same side as the gland to be removed, while the scrub nurse is on the opposite side. The screen is positioned directly in front of the surgeon, at eye level. The surgeon utilizes both working ports, and the scopist is responsible for manipulating the camera throughout the procedure [41].

5.2. Trocar Placement Technique

Proper placement of trocars is essential in retroperitoneoscopic procedures. Incorrectly positioned trocars can complicate the surgery, cause discomfort and strain in the surgeon's arms and back, increase anxiety in the surgical team as they struggle with instrument manipulation, and compromise patient safety. Marking anatomical landmarks prior to incision can be helpful for operative planning. As seen in Figure 6, we recommend identifying the lateral border of the paraspinous muscles, the inferior margin of the 12th rib, and the posterior superior iliac crest [24,51].

Access to the retroperitoneal space is typically gained just below the tip of the 12th rib. Key considerations during this step include avoiding injury to the pleura superiorly, identifying the correct fascial plane posterior to the kidney, and avoiding inadvertent entry into the peritoneum anteriorly. Subsequent ports are placed in a triangular configuration, with the central camera port (* in Figures 6 and 7a,b) situated 1–2 cm below the 12th rib's tip, and the two working ports placed medially (** in Figures 6 and 7a,b), bordering the paraspinous muscles, and laterally (*** in Figures 6 and 7a,b), near the posterior axillary line. An optional fourth port (blue circle in Figure 6) may be placed inferiorly for retraction if needed [24,41].

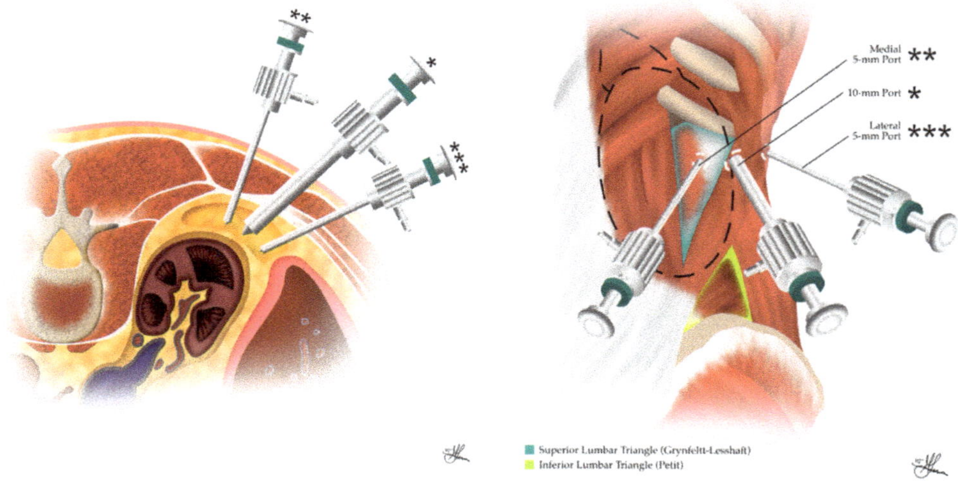

(**a**) (**b**)

Figure 7. Comparative illustrations of trocar placement for posterior retroperitoneal laparoscopic adrenalectomy on the right side: (**a**) Axial section, prone position, superior view (from the head of the patient). (**b**) Coronal section, prone position, posterior perspective (from the surgeon's perspective).

The initial 10 mm trocar insertion site is determined by palpating the 12th rib, identifying the tip of the rib, and creating a 1.5 cm transverse incision, one fingerbreadth caudally. This initial incision must admit one finger to help with blunt dissection and be able to fit a 10 mm trocar. The location of the first trocar is critical; the presence of thoracolumbar fascia rather than muscular fibers indicates an excessively medial approach (see Figure 7a). Even if the thoracolumbar fascia is encountered but the 10 mm trocar is passed just laterally to it, the superior lumbar triangle (of Grynfeltt–Lesshaft)—bound by the 12th rib superiorly, the IO muscle laterally, and the ES muscles medially (as seen in Figure 7b)—will still likely be traversed. In this thinnest area of the posterior abdominal wall, the musculo-fascial parietal anatomy, from superficial to deep, includes the latissimus dorsi muscle, EO muscle, and transversalis fascia. This region represents a potential site of reduced structural integrity in the posterior abdominal wall. While direct traversal of this triangle is not contraindicated, it necessitates meticulous closure to mitigate the risk of incisional hernia formation. Conversely, the optimal trajectory traverses the skin, subcutaneous adipose tissue, and EO, IO, and TA muscles, in that order, culminating in the penetration of the transversalis fascia to access the retroperitoneum, i.e., the posterior pararenal space (see Figure 5). Therefore, encountering the latissimus dorsi indicates that the incision is placed too supero-medial [24,32,41].

Access to the retroperitoneal space is accomplished by blunt dissection with a Kelly clamp or sharp dissection with scissors. Once retroperitoneal access is achieved, a finger sweep should be performed, with further blind blunt digital dissection extended medially and laterally, to allow for the creation of sufficient retroperitoneal space for the insertion of two more 5 mm work trocars. With an index finger inserted into the retroperitoneal space, guiding the insertion just lateral to the paraspinous muscles, approximately 3 cm below the 12th rib, the first 5 mm medial trocar is carefully positioned, angled cranially at 45 degrees to optimize access to the surgical field. Similarly, positioned 4–5 cm lateral to the initial incision, below the 11th rib, the second 5 mm lateral trocar is inserted. Finally, a larger 10–12 mm blunt trocar, equipped with an inflatable dissector balloon, is passed through the initial incision site and serves as the main working port for the procedure.

Once all ports are successfully positioned, the surgeon establishes pneumoretroperitoneum by insufflating the retroperitoneal space with CO_2 gas. The pressure is carefully maintained between 20 and 28 mmHg, creating and sustaining the necessary working space for the adrenalectomy in the relatively non-compliant retroperitoneal cavity [41,52].

Alternatively, following initial access, the creation of a sufficient working space within the retroperitoneum is achieved through either digital dissection or the direct deployment of a balloon dissector. After the first 10 mm trocar is inserted and secured, pneumoretroperitoneum is then established from the beginning, and a 30° laparoscope is passed, aiding with further blunt dissection. Finally, in the same positions as described above, but under direct laparoscopic visualization, the two additional 5 mm trocars are inserted. The lateral port is placed a minimum of 3 cm from the central port to minimize instrument interference while maintaining triangulation [25]. The resulting trocar configuration forms a horizontal alignment, which allows for dynamic adaptation of the port function intraoperatively, facilitating optimal visualization and instrument maneuverability in response to individual anatomical variations and specific surgical challenges.

5.3. Workspace Development

Creating an adequate retroperitoneal workspace can be the most challenging task in PRLA. As stated above, patient positioning is essential for allowing this to occur. With the abdominal contents hanging freely, the retroperitoneal cavity is expanded, in the prone jackknife position. However, the working space can differ between sides. The right side often provides a slightly more confined working area due to the presence of the liver, while the left side may offer more room for manipulation, particularly in the upper pole of the gland. Another key difference lies in the surrounding structures that must be navigated. On the right, the liver serves as an important landmark and potential obstacle, while on the left, the spleen and pancreatic tail are the primary structures of concern. The right-sided procedure often requires more careful retraction of the liver to obtain adequate exposure [53].

Regardless of the trocar placement technique, initially, a 10 mm 30° endoscope is introduced through the middle trocar. This larger scope is used to begin the creation of the retroperitoneal space. The surgeon employs a combination of blunt and sharp dissection techniques to carefully expand this area, providing the necessary room for the procedure. Once this initial space is established, the surgeon transitions to a smaller, more maneuverable instrument. The 10 mm scope is replaced with a 5 mm 30-degree scope, which is then inserted through the medial trocar. This change allows for greater flexibility and improved visualization in the confined retroperitoneal space [52].

With the 5 mm scope in place, the surgeon focuses on expanding the retroperitoneal space beneath the diaphragm. This is achieved by applying downward pressure on the fatty tissue in this area. The goal is to create sufficient working space while maintaining careful control to avoid injury to surrounding structures.

A key step in this process is the identification of and entry into Gerota's fascia. This fascial layer encapsulates the kidney and the adrenal gland, and its careful dissection is crucial for accessing the adrenal gland. As the dissection progresses, the surgeon works to identify the superior pole of the kidney. This anatomical landmark serves as a critical reference point during the procedure. Locating the superior pole of the kidney not only helps orient the surgeon within the retroperitoneal space but also guides the subsequent dissection towards the adrenal gland, which is typically located just above and medial to this point. This meticulous approach to creating and navigating the retroperitoneal space sets the stage for the subsequent steps of the adrenalectomy, ensuring optimal visibility and access to the adrenal gland while minimizing the risk of injury to surrounding structures [41,52].

As the dissection progresses deeper, the surgeon encounters the paraspinous muscles and, ultimately, visualizes the adrenal gland. The anatomical landscape differs slightly between the right and left sides. On the right, the IVC serves as a crucial anatomical reference point, and it is not uncommon to glimpse the liver through the translucent posterior peritoneum. In contrast, when operating on the left side, the spleen or the posterior gastric wall may be visible through the thin peritoneal lining [41]. These surrounding structures provide important spatial orientation during the procedure, guiding the surgeon's approach to the adrenal gland.

6. Optimal Approach to Adrenal Dissection

The PRLA technique, while similar in overall approach, presents distinct challenges and considerations depending on whether the left or right adrenal gland is being addressed. Understanding these differences is crucial for optimal surgical outcomes.

For both sides, the initial steps are similar: patient positioning in a prone jackknife position, trocar placement, and creation of the retroperitoneal space. Dissection commences at the inferior pole of the adrenal gland, progressing medially. Small arterial vessels feeding the gland are divided using electrocautery, i.e., vascular sealing devices. It is crucial to maintain the superior attachments of the adrenal gland intact at this stage, allowing it to "hang" and facilitating further dissection [52]. This strategy minimizes manipulation of the relatively fragile adrenal tissue. However, as the dissection progresses, key anatomical differences become apparent.

On the right side, dissection begins lateral and posterior to the right lobe of the liver, progressing medially until the lateral aspect of the IVC is visualized. The right adrenal vein, a critical structure, is typically found posterolateral to the IVC, often close to the diaphragm. It courses medially to drain directly into the IVC (see Figure 8a,b). The surgeon must exercise extreme caution when dissecting in this area, as inadvertent injury to the IVC can lead to significant bleeding. The high insufflation pressure used in PRLA often flattens the IVC, causing it to lose its tubular appearance and appear as a white line along its lateral border [24,25,41,54].

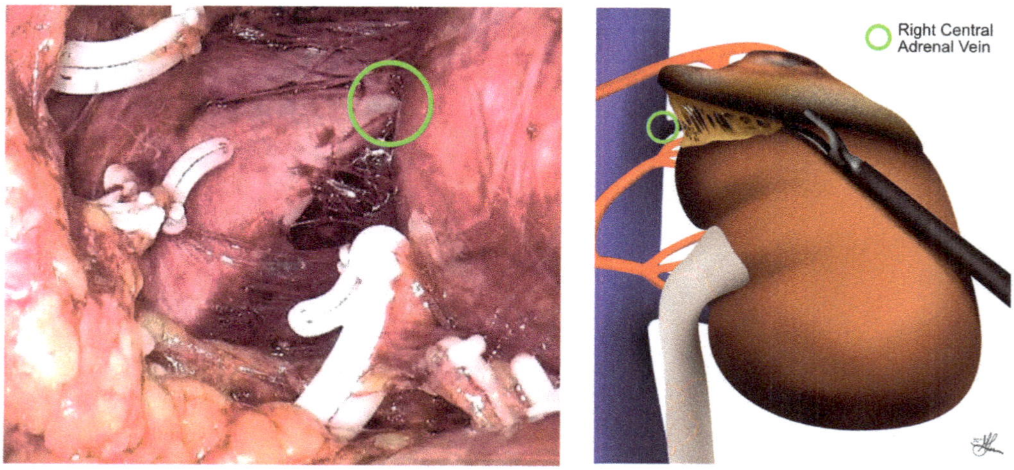

(a) (b)

Figure 8. Right posterior retroperitoneal laparoscopic adrenalectomy, with the characteristic junction between the central right adrenal vein and the inferior vena cava highlighted by the green circle: (**a**) live surgery image; (**b**) illustration.

In contrast, left-sided adrenalectomy presents a different set of anatomical relationships. Dissection on the left begins laterally, in the plane between the kidney and the adrenal gland, behind the spleen. As dissection continues medially, the surgeon must be aware of the proximity of the pancreatic tail and take care to avoid injury. The left adrenal vein is typically found medial to the upper pole of the kidney, draining inferiorly into the left renal vein, usually within a common venous trunk formed by its junction with the left inferior phrenic vein superiorly (see Figure 9a,b), rather than directly into the IVC as on the right side. This anatomical arrangement often makes the left adrenal vein easier to identify and control [24,25,41,54].

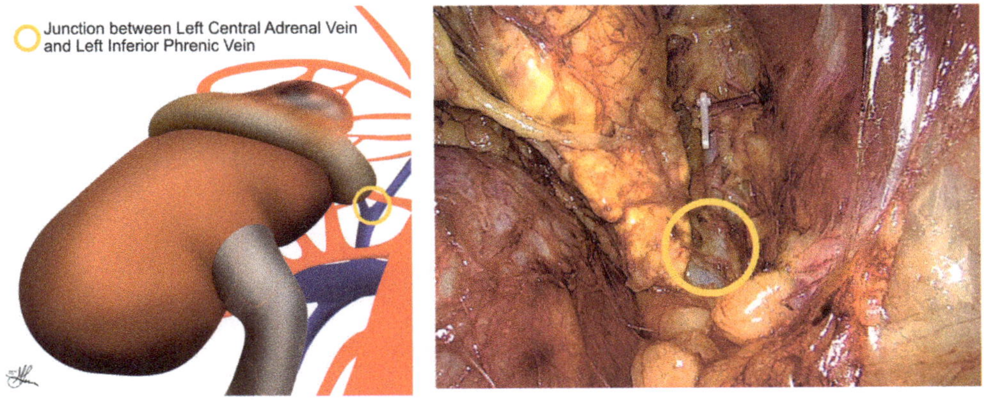

(a) (b)

Figure 9. Left posterior retroperitoneal laparoscopic adrenalectomy, with the characteristic junction between the central left adrenal vein and the left inferior phrenic vein highlighted by the yellow circle: (**a**) illustration; (**b**) live surgery image.

Overall, in terms of the adrenal vein management, while both sides require careful isolation and ligation, the right adrenal vein is often shorter and more challenging to dissect due to its proximity to the IVC. On the left, the adrenal vein is typically longer and more easily isolated, but care must be taken not to injure the left renal vein during dissection. Thus, on both sides, once identified, the adrenal vein should be circumferentially dissected for about 1 cm and ligated using an advanced sealing device or clips. This step is crucial for maintaining hemostasis and preventing inadvertent bleeding. After securing the adrenal vein, dissection continues laterally and superiorly. The adrenal vein's stump can be used as a handle for manipulation, minimizing direct grasping of the friable adrenal tissue. The phrenic vein may be divided if needed but can often be preserved. For both sides, small arterial branches are encountered and coagulated throughout the dissection. However, the right side may require more meticulous dissection due to the presence of small arteries crossing the IVC posteriorly [24,25,41,54].

Adrenal gland dissection is completed by freeing the gland from its remaining attachments to the paraspinous muscles and peritoneum. Throughout this process, it is important to avoid grasping the actual adrenal parenchyma, which is easily fractured. Once fully mobilized, the specimen is placed in a retrieval bag and extracted through the middle trocar site, which may occasionally need minimal enlargement. Before closure, the insufflation pressure is reduced to 8–12 mmHg to check for any venous bleeding that might have been tamponaded by the high CO_2 pressure. The adrenal bed is irrigated, and meticulous hemostasis is achieved. Lastly, the trocar insertion sites must be checked for bleeding after trocar removal, and the incisions must be closed appropriately. The fascia of the 10 mm trocar site should ideally be closed with a figure-of-eight suture, and the skin of all port sites with a subcuticular stitch [41,54].

Importantly, throughout the procedure, vigilance must be maintained against potential complications such as pneumothorax or peritoneal breach, which could lead to inadvertent injury of adjacent organs, i.e., the spleen, pancreas, or liver. A chest X-ray in the recovery area can ensure that no pneumothorax has occurred.

This systematic approach to PRLA, coupled with the surgeon's growing experience in identifying the bright yellow appearance of the adrenal cortex amid retroperitoneal fat, ensures safe and effective adrenal gland removal while minimizing the risk of complications. The high-pressure pneumoretroperitoneum not only creates additional working space in this confined area but also helps to tamponade minor bleeding from small arterioles, contributing to the procedure's efficiency and safety.

7. Surgical Tips and Tricks

PRLA has emerged as a safe, fast, and effective procedure with a low complication rate. However, mastering this technique requires attention to several key aspects and potential challenges. This section provides a comprehensive overview of essential tips and tricks to optimize the surgical approach and outcomes.

One of the initial concerns with PRLA was the ability to create adequate working space in the retroperitoneum using traditional insufflation pressures. Contrary to early apprehensions about higher insufflation pressures decreasing venous return and causing hypotension due to IVC compression, research has demonstrated that patients maintain normal cardiac output and filling pressures with elevated retroperitoneal insufflation levels. Studies comparing intra- and extra-thoracic IVC pressures during laparoscopic cholecystectomy and PRLA revealed that while cardiac filling decreased with intraperitoneal insufflation pressures above 15 mmHg, it remained stable with retroperitoneal insufflation pressures exceeding this threshold. Consequently, surgeons can safely use higher insufflation pressures (up to 28–30 mmHg) to create sufficient working space and achieve a relatively bloodless operative field [54].

In obese patients (BMI > 35), increasing retroperitoneal pneumo-insufflation up to 30 mmHg can help establish an adequate working space. However, patients with a BMI > 45 may not be ideal candidates for PRLA. In these cases, the compression of the retroperitoneum by abdominal organs in the prone position can make it extremely challenging to create sufficient space, even with high insufflation pressures. Some studies have reported the need to convert to a transabdominal approach in patients with BMI > 45 due to this issue. While obesity does not preclude PRLA, it does make the procedure more technically challenging and time-consuming, underscoring the importance of careful patient selection and surgeon experience [41].

Correct trocar placement is crucial for safe and comfortable gland dissection. The trocars should be placed at an acute angle towards the adrenal. This becomes even more critical in obese patients or in males with thick muscle walls. In rare instances of trocar misplacement causing pleural tears, the procedure can often be continued by sealing the leakage with a blunt-tipped trocar with a balloon and inserting a pleural drain until the end of the operation. If the peritoneal cavity is inadvertently entered during the procedure, surgery can typically still be completed using the posterior retroperitoneoscopic approach without additional intervention, as there is no compression of the retroperitoneum by the abdominal viscera [55].

Identifying the upper pole of the kidney is paramount, as it provides the critical anatomical landmark for safe progression of the procedure [56,57]. Dissection should always proceed from "lateral to medial" and from "bottom to top", commencing at the lower pole of the suprarenal gland. Right-sided dissection should follow a clockwise movement from 3 to 9 o'clock, while on the left side it should be counterclockwise from 9 to 3 o'clock. This approach helps avoid injury to the renal vessels [17]. The left adrenal gland's position, falling in front of the superior part of the left kidney's anterior surface, necessitates extended kidney mobilization for complete gland resection. This can be achieved by applying pressure on the kidney's upper pole with a non-traumatic grasper.

Retroperitoneal fatty tissue can significantly obscure the surgical field, especially in obese patients or those with Cushing's syndrome. Removing this tissue, often possible through suctioning, especially around the superior renal pole and its ipsilateral adrenal, can help expose crucial anatomical landmarks [58]. This step is essential for identifying key structures and facilitating safe dissection [54].

Vascular considerations are critical in PRLA. The right adrenal vein, typically short and positioned behind the gland and in front of the IVC, can be challenging to locate and dissect. Gently lifting the right adrenal from the IVC can create a small fold on the IVC's dorsal surface, helping to locate the vein. When dissecting near the IVC, using a "pinch and pull" technique on fatty tissue can help ensure that the vein is not inadvertently grasped. Ligating the medial adrenal arteries crossing the vena cava in a retro-caval position may aid in exposing the IVC [17].

While significant bleeding is rare in PRLA, it can usually be controlled by the 20–25 mmHg pressure and energy devices. Applying compression with gauze is often the fastest and simplest way to control bleeding if it occurs. Clips can be used cautiously if needed, but they are rarely necessary. The high CO_2 pressure in the retroperitoneal space helps to tamponade small-vessel bleeding, contributing to the procedure's safety.

Managing potential complications is an essential aspect of PRLA. Pneumothorax can occur if the pleural space is violated during trocar placement or dissection, with reported rates between <1 and 3.4%. Palpable subcutaneous emphysema may also occur but is typically asymptomatic and does not alter the hospital course. Rarely, a fourth trocar may be placed below the line of the first trocars (see Figure 6). This additional port may be useful in placing a vascular clamp to control bleeding in the event of a major vascular injury, or for kidney retraction in obese patients [54].

During the procedure, keeping the left adrenal vein grasped with a non-traumatic grasper after ligation can help mobilize the gland throughout the remaining procedure, without capsule rupture [59]. This technique is not applicable to the short right adrenal vein. When dissecting the entire gland, dissecting from "top to bottom" may occasionally help to mobilize it completely [54,55].

PRLA is a technically demanding procedure that requires a thorough understanding of the retroperitoneal anatomy. With experience and proper technique, it offers a safe and effective approach for adrenal surgery, even in challenging cases. However, careful patient selection, especially regarding BMI, remains crucial for optimal outcomes. As with any advanced laparoscopic procedure, the learning curve can be significant, and surgeons should ideally gain experience under the guidance of an experienced mentor before attempting complex cases independently.

8. Conclusions

In conclusion, PRLA represents a significant advancement in the field of adrenal surgery, offering numerous benefits over traditional open approaches. Its adoption has been driven by the clear advantages of reduced postoperative pain, shorter hospital stays, faster recovery times, and comparable long-term outcomes. However, the expertise of the surgical team and the specific characteristics of each case must guide the choice of surgical approach, as PRLA is not without limitations. Obesity, large tumors, and suspected malignancies may pose significant challenges or contraindications. With careful patient selection, meticulous perioperative management, and a multidisciplinary approach, PRLA provides an effective and minimally invasive option for treating adrenal tumors, while open surgery continues to play a crucial role in managing more complex cases. As the field of laparoscopic adrenal surgery continues to evolve, further research and advancements in techniques and technology will likely expand the indications and improve outcomes for patients undergoing this innovative procedure.

Author Contributions: Conceptualization, B.O.F., V.B., S.C.L., A.B. and D.N.; methodology, B.O.F., A.A.C. and D.P.-H.; software, C.-S.D. and V.B.; validation, T.G.C., A.C.B. and D.N.; formal analysis, C.-S.D., A.A.C. and A.C.B.; investigation, B.O.F., A.B. and D.P.-H.; resources, C.-S.D., T.G.C., V.B. and D.P.-H.; data curation, A.C.B., A.B., F.Z. and H.I.; writing—original draft preparation, B.O.F., V.B. and D.N.; writing—review and editing S.C.L., H.I., F.Z. and T.G.C.; visualization, F.Z., A.A.C., H.I.

and S.C.L.; supervision, D.N.; project administration, D.N.; funding acquisition, not applicable. All authors have read and agreed to the published version of the manuscript.

Funding: We would like to acknowledge Victor Babes University of Medicine and Pharmacy Timisoara for their support in covering the costs of publication for this research paper.

Data Availability Statement: Data are available upon request.

Acknowledgments: We, the authors, would like to thank our very talented graphic designer, Marius Filip, for his invaluable contributions to the current paper.

Conflicts of Interest: The authors declare no conflicts of interest.

References

1. Uludağ, M.; Aygün, N.; İşgör, A. Surgical Indications and Techniques for Adrenalectomy. *Sisli Etfal Hastan. Tip. Bul.* **2020**, *54*, 8–22. [CrossRef] [PubMed]
2. Prager, G.; Heinz-Peer, G.; Passler, C.; Kaczirek, K.; Schindl, M.; Scheuba, C.; Niederle, B. Surgical Strategy in Adrenal Masses. *Eur. J. Radiol.* **2002**, *41*, 70–77. [CrossRef] [PubMed]
3. Matsuda, T. Laparoscopic Adrenalectomy: The "gold Standard" When Performed Appropriately. *BJU Int.* **2017**, *119*, 2–3. [CrossRef] [PubMed]
4. Go, H.; Takeda, M.; Takahashi, H.; Imai, T.; Tsutsui, T.; Mizusawa, T.; Nishiyama, T.; Morishita, H.; Nakajima, Y.; Sato, S. Laparoscopic Adrenalectomy for Primary Aldosteronism: A New Operative Method. *J. Laparoendosc. Surg.* **1993**, *3*, 455–459. [CrossRef]
5. Higashihara, E.; Tanaka, Y.; Horie, S.; Aruga, S.; Nutahara, K.; Homma, Y.; Minowada, S.; Aso, Y. A case report of laparoscopic adrenalectomy. *Nihon Hinyokika Gakkai Zasshi* **1992**, *83*, 1130–1133. [CrossRef]
6. Gagner, M.; Lacroix, A.; Bolté, E. Laparoscopic Adrenalectomy in Cushing's Syndrome and Pheochromocytoma. *N. Engl. J. Med.* **1992**, *327*, 1033. [CrossRef]
7. Wu, C.-T.; Chiang, Y.-J.; Chou, C.-C.; Liu, K.-L.; Lee, S.-H.; Chang, Y.-H.; Chuang, C.-K. Comparative Study of Laparoscopic and Open Adrenalectomy. *Chang. Gung Med. J.* **2005**, *29*, 468–473.
8. Al-Jalabneh, T.; Al-Shawabkeh, O.; Al-Gwairy, I.; Abu-Zeitoun, O.; Al-Njadat, I.; Al-Soudi, M.; Zarour, A. Laparoscopic Versus Open Adrenalectomy: A Retrospective Comparative Study. *Med. Arch.* **2021**, *75*, 41–44. [CrossRef]
9. Guerrieri, M.; Campagnacci, R.; De Sanctis, A.; Baldarelli, M.; Coletta, M.; Perretta, S. The Learning Curve in Laparoscopic Adrenalectomy. *J. Endocrinol. Investig.* **2008**, *31*, 531–536. [CrossRef]
10. Guidelines for the Minimally Invasive Treatment of Adrenal Pathology—A SAGES Publication. SAGES. Available online: https://www.sages.org/publications/guidelines/guidelines-for-the-minimally-invasive-treatment-of-adrenal-pathology/ (accessed on 25 September 2024).
11. Kapoor, A.; Morris, T.; Rebello, R. Guidelines for the Management of the Incidentally Discovered Adrenal Mass. *Can. Urol. Assoc. J.* **2011**, *5*, 241–247. [CrossRef]
12. Tanaka, M.; Ono, Y.; Matsuda, T.; Terachi, T.; Suzuki, K.; Baba, S.; Hara, I.; Hirao, Y.; Urological Laparoscopic Surgery Guideline Committee, Japanese Society of Endourology and ESWL. Guidelines for Urological Laparoscopic Surgery. *Int. J. Urol.* **2009**, *16*, 115–125. [CrossRef] [PubMed]
13. Maccora, D.; Walls, G.; Sadler, G.; Mihai, R. Bilateral Adrenalectomy: A Review of 10 Years' Experience. *Ann. R. Coll. Surg. Engl.* **2017**, *99*, 119–122. [CrossRef] [PubMed]
14. Mercan, S.; Seven, R.; Ozarmagan, S.; Tezelman, S. Endoscopic Retroperitoneal Adrenalectomy. *Surgery* **1995**, *118*, 1071–1075; discussion 1075–1076. [CrossRef] [PubMed]
15. Walz, M.K.; Peitgen, K.; Hoermann, R.; Giebler, R.M.; Mann, K.; Eigler, F.W. Posterior Retroperitoneoscopy as a New Minimally Invasive Approach for Adrenalectomy: Results of 30 Adrenalectomies in 27 Patients. *World J. Surg.* **1996**, *20*, 769–774. [CrossRef] [PubMed]
16. Mihai, R. Bilateral Adrenalectomy—Simultaneous or Delayed? *Laparosc. Surg.* **2019**, *3*. [CrossRef]
17. Alesina, P.F. Retroperitoneal Adrenalectomy—Learning Curve, Practical Tips and Tricks, What Limits Its Wider Uptake. *Gland. Surg.* **2019**, *8* (Suppl. 1), S36–S40. [CrossRef]
18. Walz, M.K.; Alesina, P.F.; Wenger, F.A.; Deligiannis, A.; Szuczik, E.; Petersenn, S.; Ommer, A.; Groeben, H.; Peitgen, K.; Janssen, O.E.; et al. Posterior Retroperitoneoscopic Adrenalectomy—Results of 560 Procedures in 520 Patients. *Surgery* **2006**, *140*, 943–948; discussion 948–950. [CrossRef]
19. Chai, Y.J.; Yu, H.W.; Song, R.-Y.; Kim, S.; Choi, J.Y.; Lee, K.E. Lateral Transperitoneal Adrenalectomy Versus Posterior Retroperitoneoscopic Adrenalectomy for Benign Adrenal Gland Disease: Randomized Controlled Trial at a Single Tertiary Medical Center. *Ann. Surg.* **2019**, *269*, 842. [CrossRef]
20. Jiang, Y.-L.; Qian, L.-J.; Li, Z.; Wang, K.-E.; Zhou, X.-L.; Zhou, J.; Ye, C.-H. Comparison of the Retroperitoneal versus Transperitoneal Laparoscopic Adrenalectomy Perioperative Outcomes and Safety for Pheochromocytoma: A Meta-Analysis. *BMC Surg.* **2020**, *20*, 12. [CrossRef]

21. Alemanno, G.; Bergamini, C.; Prosperi, P.; Valeri, A. Adrenalectomy: Indications and Options for Treatment. *Updates Surg.* **2017**, *69*, 119–125. [CrossRef]
22. Lal, G.; Clark, O.H. Thyroid, Parathyroid, and Adrenal. In *Schwartz's Principles of Surgery*; Brunicardi, F.C., Andersen, D.K., Billiar, T.R., Dunn, D.L., Kao, L.S., Hunter, J.G., Matthews, J.B., Pollock, R.E., Eds.; McGraw-Hill Education: New York, NY, USA, 2019.
23. Mihai, I.; Boicean, A.; Teodoru, C.A.; Grigore, N.; Iancu, G.M.; Dura, H.; Bratu, D.G.; Roman, M.D.; Mohor, C.I.; Todor, S.B.; et al. Laparoscopic Adrenalectomy: Tailoring Approaches for the Optimal Resection of Adrenal Tumors. *Diagnostics* **2023**, *13*, 3351. [CrossRef] [PubMed]
24. Fuentes, M.B.; Keat, C.W. Laparoscopic Adrenalectomy: Retroperitoneal Approach. In *Mastering Endo-Laparoscopic and Thoracoscopic Surgery: ELSA Manual*; Lomanto, D., Chen, W.T.-L., Fuentes, M.B., Eds.; Springer Nature: Singapore, 2023; pp. 161–165. [CrossRef]
25. McCoy, K.; Valdez, C.; Gibson, C.E. Retroperitoneoscopic Adrenalectomy: Indications and Technical Considerations. *Laparosc. Surg.* **2022**, *6*. [CrossRef]
26. Lenders, J.W.M.; Duh, Q.-Y.; Eisenhofer, G.; Gimenez-Roqueplo, A.-P.; Grebe, S.K.G.; Murad, M.H.; Naruse, M.; Pacak, K.; Young, W.F.; Endocrine Society. Pheochromocytoma and Paraganglioma: An Endocrine Society Clinical Practice Guideline. *J. Clin. Endocrinol. Metab.* **2014**, *99*, 1915–1942. [CrossRef] [PubMed]
27. Arezzo, A.; Bullano, A.; Cochetti, G.; Cirocchi, R.; Randolph, J.; Mearini, E.; Evangelista, A.; Ciccone, G.; Bonjer, H.J.; Morino, M. Transperitoneal versus Retroperitoneal Laparoscopic Adrenalectomy for Adrenal Tumours in Adults. *Cochrane Database Syst. Rev.* **2018**, *2018*, CD011668. [CrossRef] [PubMed]
28. Berruti, A.; Baudin, E.; Gelderblom, H.; Haak, H.R.; Porpiglia, F.; Fassnacht, M.; Pentheroudakis, G.; ESMO Guidelines Working Group. Adrenal Cancer: ESMO Clinical Practice Guidelines for Diagnosis, Treatment and Follow-Up. *Ann. Oncol.* **2012**, *23* (Suppl. 7), vii131–vii138. [CrossRef]
29. Fassnacht, M.; Dekkers, O.; Else, T.; Baudin, E.; Berruti, A.; de Krijger, R.; Haak, H.; Mihai, R.; Assie, G.; Terzolo, M. European Society of Endocrinology Clinical Practice Guidelines on the Management of Adrenocortical Carcinoma in Adults, in Collaboration with the European Network for the Study of Adrenal Tumors. *Eur. J. Endocrinol.* **2018**, *179*, G1–G46. [CrossRef]
30. Gaujoux, S.; Mihai, R.; joint working group of ESES and ENSAT. European Society of Endocrine Surgeons (ESES) and European Network for the Study of Adrenal Tumours (ENSAT) Recommendations for the Surgical Management of Adrenocortical Carcinoma. *Br. J. Surg.* **2017**, *104*, 358–376. [CrossRef]
31. Callender, G.G.; Kennamer, D.L.; Grubbs, E.G.; Lee, J.E.; Evans, D.B.; Perrier, N.D. Posterior Retroperitoneoscopic Adrenalectomy. *Adv. Surg.* **2009**, *43*, 147–157. [CrossRef]
32. Caroço, T.V.; Costa Almeida, C.E. Anatomy of the Adrenal Gland. In *Posterior Retroperitoneoscopic Adrenalectomy: Indications, Technical Steps and Outcomes*; Eduardo Costa Almeida, C., Ed.; Springer International Publishing: Cham, Switzerland, 2023; pp. 1–9. [CrossRef]
33. Ceccato, F.; Scaroni, C.; Boscaro, M. The Adrenal Glands. In *Principles of Endocrinology and Hormone Action*; Belfiore, A., LeRoith, D., Eds.; Springer International Publishing: Cham, Switzerland, 2016; pp. 1–35. [CrossRef]
34. Van Slycke, S.; Van Den Heede, K.; Vandenwyngaerden, E.-A. Adrenal Glands: Anatomy, Physiology, and Pathophysiology. In *Endocrine Surgery Comprehensive Board Exam Guide*; Shifrin, A.L., Raffaelli, M., Randolph, G.W., Gimm, O., Eds.; Springer International Publishing: Cham, Switzerland, 2021; pp. 437–455. [CrossRef]
35. Clark, O.H.; Duh, Q.-Y.; Kebebew, E.; Gosnell, J.E.; Shen, W.T. Textbook of Endocrine Surgery. JP Medical Ltd.: New Delhi, India, 2016.
36. Avisse, C.; Marcus, C.; Patey, M.; Ladam-Marcus, V.; Delattre, J.F.; Flament, J.B. Surgical Anatomy and Embryology of the Adrenal Glands. *Surg. Clin. North. Am.* **2000**, *80*, 403–415. [CrossRef]
37. Feigelson, B.J. Adrenal Glands. In *Surgical Anatomy and Technique: A Pocket Manual*; Skandalakis, L.J., Ed.; Springer International Publishing: Cham, Switzerland, 2021; pp. 673–699. [CrossRef]
38. Themes, U.F.O. The Adrenal Glands. Thoracic Key. Available online: https://thoracickey.com/the-adrenal-glands/ (accessed on 26 September 2024).
39. Cesmebasi, A.; Du Plessis, M.; Iannatuono, M.; Shah, S.; Tubbs, R.S.; Loukas, M. A Review of the Anatomy and Clinical Significance of Adrenal Veins. *Clin. Anat.* **2014**, *27*, 1253–1263. [CrossRef]
40. Megha, R.; Wehrle, C.J.; Kashyap, S.; Leslie, S.W. Anatomy, Abdomen and Pelvis: Adrenal Glands (Suprarenal Glands). In *StatPearls*; StatPearls Publishing: Treasure Island, FL, USA, 2024.
41. Costa Almeida, C.E. Technical Steps of Posterior Retroperitoneoscopic Adrenalectomy. In *Posterior Retroperitoneoscopic Adrenalectomy: Indications, Technical Steps and Outcomes*; Eduardo Costa Almeida, C., Ed.; Springer International Publishing: Cham, Switzerland, 2023; pp. 59–70. [CrossRef]
42. Flynn, W.; Vickerton, P. Anatomy, Abdomen and Pelvis: Abdominal Wall. In *StatPearls*; StatPearls Publishing: Treasure Island, FL, USA, 2024.
43. Loukas, M.; El-Zammar, D.; Shoja, M.; Tubbs, R.S.; Zhan, L.; Protyniak, B.; Krutoshinskaya, Y. The Clinical Anatomy of the Triangle of Grynfeltt. *Hernia J. Hernias Abdom. Wall Surg.* **2008**, *12*, 227–231. [CrossRef] [PubMed]
44. Armstrong, O.; Hamel, A.; Grignon, B.; NDoye, J.M.; Hamel, O.; Robert, R.; Rogez, J.M. Lumbar Hernia: Anatomical Basis and Clinical Aspects. *Surg. Radiol. Anat.* **2008**, *30*, 533–537; discussion 609–610. [CrossRef] [PubMed]
45. Orcutt, T.W. Hernia of the Superior Lumbar Triangle. *Ann. Surg.* **1971**, *173*, 294–297. [CrossRef] [PubMed]

46. Standring, S. *Gray's Anatomy: The Anatomical Basis of Clinical Practice*; Elsevier: Amsterdam, The Netherlands, 2020.
47. Tirkes, T.; Sandrasegaran, K.; Patel, A.A.; Hollar, M.A.; Tejada, J.G.; Tann, M.; Akisik, F.M.; Lappas, J.C. Peritoneal an Retroperitoneal Anatomy and Its Relevance for Cross-Sectional Imaging. *Radiographics* **2012**, *32*, 437–451. [CrossRef] [PubMed
48. Raslau, D.; Bierle, D.M.; Stephenson, C.R.; Mikhail, M.A.; Kebede, E.B.; Mauck, K.F. Preoperative Cardiac Risk Assessment. *Ma Clin. Proc.* **2020**, *95*, 1064–1079. [CrossRef]
49. Edgcombe, H.; Carter, K.; Yarrow, S. Anaesthesia in the Prone Position. *Br. J. Anaesth.* **2008**, *100*, 165–183. [CrossRef]
50. Feltracco, P.; Barbieri, S.; Carron, M. Anesthesia in Posterior Retroperitoneoscopic Approach. In *Posterior Retroperitoneoscop Adrenalectomy: Indications, Technical Steps and Outcomes*; Eduardo Costa Almeida, C., Ed.; Springer International Publishing: Char Switzerland, 2023; pp. 49–58. [CrossRef]
51. Themes, U.F.O. Minimally Invasive Retroperitoneal Adrenalectomy. Abdominal Key. Available online: https://abdominalke com/minimally-invasive-retroperitoneal-adrenalectomy/ (accessed on 26 September 2024).
52. Cayo, A.K.; Wang, T.S. Laparoscopic Adrenalectomy: Retroperitoneal Approach. *Curr. Surg. Rep.* **2013**, *1*, 34–39. [CrossRef]
53. Themes, U.F.O. Posterior Retroperitoneoscopic Adrenalectomy. Oncohema Key. Available online: https://oncohemakey.com posterior-retroperitoneoscopic-adrenalectomy/ (accessed on 26 September 2024).
54. Walz, M.K. Posterior Retroperitoneoscopic Adrenalectomy. In *Adrenal Glands*; Linos, D., Van Heerden, J.A., Eds.; Springe Berlin/Heidelberg, Germany, 2005; pp. 333–339. [CrossRef]
55. Perrier, N.D.; Kennamer, D.L.; Bao, R.; Jimenez, C.; Grubbs, E.G.; Lee, J.E.; Evans, D.B. Posterior Retroperitoneoscopic Adrenale tomy: Preferred Technique for Removal of Benign Tumors and Isolated Metastases. *Ann. Surg.* **2008**, *248*, 666–674. [CrossRef]
56. Grosso, A.A.; Di Maida, F.; Tellini, R.; Mari, A.; Sforza, S.; Masieri, L.; Carini, M.; Minervini, A. Robot-Assisted Partia Nephrectomy with 3D Preoperative Surgical Planning: Video Presentation of the Florentine Experience. *Int. Braz. J. Urol.* **2021**, *47* 1272–1273. [CrossRef]
57. Grosso, A.A.; Di Maida, F.; Lambertini, L.; Cadenar, A.; Coco, S.; Ciaralli, E.; Salamone, V.; Vittori, G.; Tuccio, A.; Mari, A. et al. Three-Dimensional Virtual Model for Robot-Assisted Partial Nephrectomy: A Propensity-Score Matching Analysis with a Contemporary Control Group. *World J. Urol.* **2024**, *42*, 338. [CrossRef]
58. Simone, G.; Anceschi, U.; Tuderti, G.; Misuraca, L.; Celia, A.; De Concilio, B.; Costantini, M.; Stigliano, A.; Minisola, F.; Ferriero M.; et al. Robot-Assisted Partial Adrenalectomy for the Treatment of Conn's Syndrome: Surgical Technique, and Perioperative and Functional Outcomes. *Eur. Urol.* **2019**, *75*, 811–816. [CrossRef]
59. Ferriero, M.; Iannuzzi, A.; Bove, A.M.; Tuderti, G.; Anceschi, U.; Misuraca, L.; Brassetti, A.; Mastroianni, R.; Guaglianone, S. Leonardo, C.; et al. Adrenalectomy for Metastasis: The Impact of Primary Histology on Survival Outcome. *Cancers* **2024**, *16*, 763 [CrossRef]

cancers

MDPI

Article

Minimally Invasive One-Docking, Two-Target, and Three-Port Robotic-Assisted Nephroureterectomy: Redefining Surgical Approach

Yarden Zohar, Ben Hefer, Itay Vazana, Muhammad H. Jabareen, Rabea Moed, Elad Mazor, Emilio Charabati, Nimer Alsaraia and Nicola J. Mabjeesh *

Department of Urology, Soroka University Medical Center, Faculty of Health Science, Ben-Gurion University of Negev, P.O. Box 151, Beer Sheva 84101, Israel; yardenzo@clalit.org.il (Y.Z.)

* Correspondence: nicolam@clalit.org.il; Tel./Fax: +972-8-6402441

Simple Summary: This study focuses on robotic radical nephroureterectomy performed for patients with urothelial carcinoma in their kidneys and ureters. The da Vinci Xi platform, which enhances minimally invasive surgical techniques was applied. We aimed to optimize the surgical approach by reducing the number of ports used, and improving visualization during the procedure. The study involved 15 patients operated on by a single surgeon between 2019 and 2024, using a one docking, three-port technique. The median operative time was 133 min, and most surgeries were completed within 150 min. Blood loss was minimal, and complication rate was low. In conclusion, the study highlights that the three-port technique combined with the Xi platform is a safe and effective method for performing robotic radical nephroureterectomy, facilitating quicker procedures and achieving surgical goals.

Abstract: Objective: Nephroureterectomy (NU) is a challenging multi-quadrant surgical procedure that involves intra–infra- and retroperitoneal dissection. The introduction of the da Vinci Xi platform has further improved the minimally invasive approach. With the Xi robotic system, single docking for multi-quadrant dissection is now feasible and increasingly popular. Herein, we redefined the surgical technique by optimizing minimal port usage, maximizing template visualization, and utilizing the Xi platform's retargeting system, based on our experience with 15 patients. Methods: This single-center cohort study was based on the experience of a single surgeon with 15 patients who underwent robotic radical nephroureterectomy (RRNU) between 2019 and 2024, performed via the one docking, three-port technique. Patient data were retrospectively collected and analyzed from the medical records. Results: The cohort's median age was 79 years, with male predominance of 80%. The median operative time was 133 min, with 60% of procedures completed within 150 min; longer times (>150 min) were due to additional intraoperative non-robotic procedures. Median blood loss was 100 mL, with two patients requiring intraoperative blood transfusion. Lymph node dissection (LND) in six patients did not significantly affect the overall operative time. The intraoperative and major postoperative complication rates (Clavien-Dindo grade > III) were 13.3%. Conclusions: The use of three robotic ports combined with the Xi platform's camera-hop feature is a safe and effective technique for multi-quadrant, minimally invasive procedures, particularly in RRNU. This approach facilitates procedural goals and reduces overall operative time.

 https://doi.org/10.3390/cancers17040627

Keywords: da Vinci robotic system; multi-quadrant minimally invasive approach; nephroureterectomy; robotic single docking; three ports; robotic-assisted laparoscopic radical nephroureterectomy; robotic retargeting

1. Introduction

Radical nephroureterectomy (NU) with bladder cuff excision (BCE) is the gold-standard treatment for upper tract urothelial carcinoma (UTUC). Current guidelines indicate the importance of the surgical management of UTUC; however, there is no consensus regarding the operative approach [1]. The 'master–slave' robotic system was first introduced in the late 1990s, and the first robotic-assisted laparoscopic urology surgery was performed in 2000 [2]. Since then, the da Vinci platform has evolved. In general, the da Vinci robotic platform is superior to the laparoscopic technique owing to its 3D imaging, and the wristed configuration provides a high degree of freedom, allowing accurate and precise movements. Despite these advantages, the da Vinci platform faces limitations, including its high financial cost and economic burden, which restrict its accessibility in many public health institutions worldwide [3].

Although robot-assisted laparoscopic radical NU has already been described, its intraoperative management remains highly versatile and largely depends on surgeon experience and expertise. Standardized radical NU tetrafecta includes negative soft tissue surgical margins, BCE, lymph node dissection (LND) (for high-risk, non-metastatic disease), and no evidence of recurrence within 12 months [4,5]. The key operative goals are to minimize the overall operative time, prevent tumor seeding, and reduce the risk of urine leakage. However, the extensive nature of this surgery, especially when LND is performed, places patients at an increased risk of complications, such as major organ injury, bowel perforation, and significant blood loss. The da Vinci Xi robotic system offers distinct advantages in such complex procedures, particularly in its ability to facilitate multi-quadrant minimally invasive surgery [6]. This article presents our experience with 15 patients who underwent multi-quadrant robotic radical nephroureterectomy (RRNU) using the Xi platform. By utilizing only three ports and the camera-hop feature, we redefined the single-docking RRNU procedure to streamline the procedure and achieve favorable outcomes.

2. Patients and Methods

With the approval of the Institutional Ethics Committee, we retrospectively collected data from patients diagnosed with UTUC who underwent RRNU between 2019 and 2024. Patients who underwent NU for indications other than UTUC were excluded from the study. All patients included in the study had a suspicious lesion on imaging and were diagnosed with UTUC through diagnostic ureteroscopy (Dx URS). Following a multidisciplinary evaluation of all associated risks, they were referred for radical NU (Scheme 1). Notably, updated guidelines now allow a radical surgical approach based solely on imaging or visual appearance, without requiring biopsy-confirmed malignancy [4]. However, our study was conducted before these guideline revisions. The data included preoperative, intraoperative, and postoperative surgical details, with a follow-up period of 12 months to monitor the outcomes. All the procedures were performed by a single surgeon with up to 10 years of experience in robotic surgery. Fifteen patients met the inclusion criteria and were included in this study.

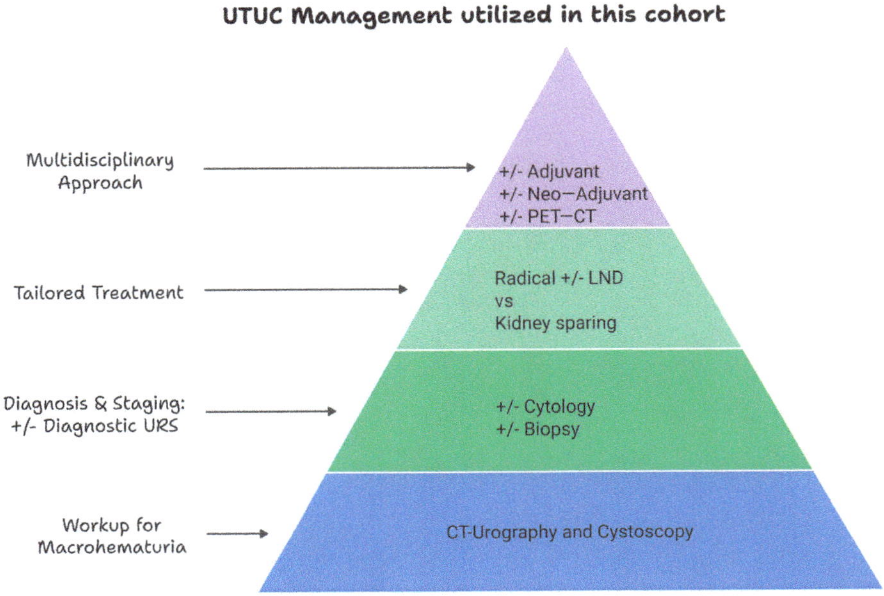

Scheme 1. Management of upper tract urothelial carcinoma (UTUC) utilized in our cohort. CT-U—computed tomography urography; LND—lymph node dissection; PET-CT—positron emission tomography–computed tomography.

3. Surgical Intervention

All 15 patients underwent RRNU with BCE by using the Xi da Vinci robotic system. The operator employed a unique intraoperative technique based on single docking for multi-quadrant surgery. After catheter insertion, patients were placed in a modified lateral decubitus position with 30-degree flexion. Trocar placement was planned along the paramedian line, with 8 cm spacing between the trocars. Three 8 mm trocars were used to dock the robotic arms, and a robotic camera was inserted through the middle port. An additional 12 mm trocar was placed in the abdominal midline, inferior to the umbilicus, and 5 cm from both the camera and the third arm trocars, forming a triangular configuration (Figure 1). The camera was initially directed toward the renal area for targeting, enabling optimal robotic arm positioning and rotation for the nephrectomy portion of the procedure.

Once docking was completed, the surgical procedure began with retroperitoneal exposure, facilitated by the dissection of Toldt's white line. After exposing the kidney, pre-renal tissue was carefully dissected and separated at the superior lateral border. After stapling the main renal blood vessels, caudal dissection was performed at the mid-ureteral level, approximately at the L2–L3 level, parallel to the gonadal vessels. Next, the assistant disconnected the robotic endpoint instruments and redirected the camera toward the pelvis. This step allowed for the retargeting of the robotic camera and reconfiguration of the robotic arms to face the pelvic area. Once the endpoint instruments were reconnected, dissection of the distal ureter was completed, and extravesical BCE was performed.

A Hem-o-lok clip was placed on the distal ureter (depending on the location of the tumor) before complete transection and separation. An inverted U-shaped stitch using a 3-0 V-Loc suture was applied at the ureteral margin to prevent urine leakage during the excision. Following the completion of the BCE procedure, the specimen was placed directly into a sealed laparoscopic bag, and the bladder was sutured with 3-0 V-Loc. In selected cases, LND was performed along the template, extending from the ipsilateral renal vein to the common iliac vessels including the external and internal iliac vessels. To minimize spillage, a separate endo-bag was used for LND specimens. A Jackson–Pratt (JP) drain was placed along the retroperitoneum from the resection bed of the kidney to the pelvis.

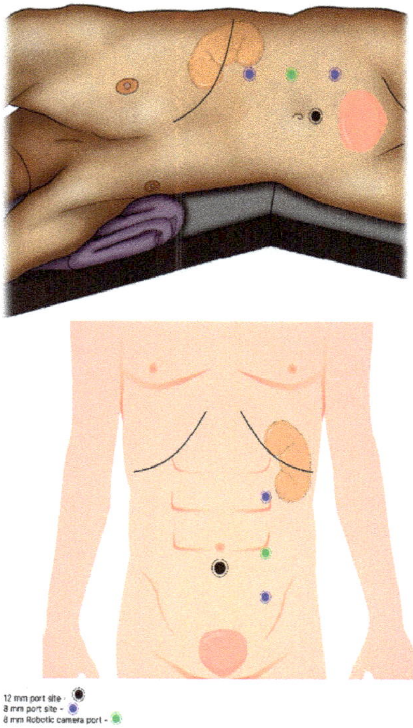

Figure 1. Patient positioning and trocar placement (black—for 12 mm trocar; blue—for 8 mm trocar; green—trocar for camera).

4. Results

Fifteen patients were included in the study, with data collected between 2019 and 2024 with a minimal follow-up period of 12 months, except for the last patient who died postoperatively. Table 1 summarizes the patients' demographic characteristics. The preoperative variables are summarized in Table 2. The median patient age was 79 years with an average age-adjusted Charlson comorbidity index score of 8.

Table 1. Demographic variables.

Total	N = 15
Age, yrs	
N	15
Mean (SD)	74.5 (9.63)
Median	79
Range	(55–86)
BMI	
Mean (SD)	26.7 (3.55)
Median	26.7
Range	21.7–33.9

Table 1. *Cont.*

Total	N = 15
Gender	
Male	12 (80%)
Female	3 (20%)
Race	
Ashkenaz Jew	10 (66.67%)
North African descent	4 (0.26%)
Other	1 (0.06%)
Age-Adjusted Charlson Comorbidity Score	
Mean	7.6
Median	8
Range	(2–14)
Personal history of cancer	
Prostate/Breast	3
Urothelial carcinoma	2
Other	1
Familial history of cancer	
Yes	7
No	2
N/A	6
Environmental exposure	
Smoking	9
Radiation	3
N/A	3
Previous abdominal surgeries	
Yes	7
No	6
N/A	2
Clinical presentation	
Hematuria	10
Back/flank pain	1
Urine retention	1
Other	3

N/A—not applicable; SD—standard deviation.

Table 2. Preoperative variables.

Total	N = 15
Hemoglobin	
Mean	12.04
Median	12
Range	7.9–15
Creatinine	
Mean	1.15
Median	1
Range	0.5–2.2
eGFR (mL/min/1.73 m^2)	
Mean	73.96
Median	66.87
Range	25.8–168.75
Oncological features	
Tumor size	
<4 cm	6
≥4 cm	9

Table 2. *Cont.*

Total	N = 15
Side	
Left	7
Right	8
Grade	
High grade	6
Low grade	8
Low grade with 5% high grade	1
Diagnostic ureteroscopy (Dx URS)	
Renal pelvis	6
Proximal ureter	3
Distal ureter	4
Orifice	2
Dx URS + TURBT	9
Neoadjuvant	
Gemcitabine/carboplatin	1
ddMVAC	1
Additional preoperative evaluation	
Renal scan (DTPA)	1
PET-CT	4
Cystoscopy (at least 1 month interval)	3

ddMVAC—dose-dense methotrexate, vinblastine, doxorubicin and cisplatin; DTPA—diethylenetriamine pentaacetate; Dx—diagnostic; PET-CT—positron emission tomography–computed tomography.

4.1. Operative Details

The median total operative time was 133 min, with 60% of the procedures completed within 150 min. Notably, LND did not significantly prolong the operative time. The median estimated blood loss (EBL) was 100 mL, with two patients requiring intraoperative blood transfusions despite controlled bleeding, attributed to their low preoperative hemoglobin levels. None of the cases required surgical technique conversion for the RRNU portion.

4.2. Lymph Node Dissection and Outcomes

LND was performed in six patients, with two showing positive nodes. Despite the extent of the procedure, no major intra- or postoperative complications were noted.

4.3. Postoperative Outcomes (Table 3)

Complications: The overall major complication rate (Clavien-Dindo grade > III) was 13.33%. One patient succumbed to cardiac arrest on postoperative day (POD) 2. Resuscitation was initiated immediately, followed by an emergency coronary angiography. Unfortunately, the last patient developed irreversible cardiac arrhythmias and did not respond to further resuscitation. The second patient was readmitted on POD 7 with type II myocardial infarction and required angioembolization.

Renal Function: The median postoperative estimated glomerular filtration rate (eGFR) was 45 mL/min/1.73 m^2, representing an average decline of 21.87 mL/min/1.73 m^2. Three patients with preoperative renal failure developed chronic renal failure (CRF). Among six patients who developed acute kidney injury postoperatively, all maintained an eGFR $\geq$ 50 mL/min/1.73 m^2 at one month.

Hospital Stay: The average hospital stay was five days. Catheters were removed on POD 3 to 5, except in one patient with bladder outlet obstruction who later underwent prostate surgery. Drains were removed on POD 4.

Table 3. Postoperative variables.

Postoperative Lab Values	(N = 15)
Hb (g/dL)	
Mean	11.2
Median	11
Range	7.5–13.9
Creatinine	
Mean	1.6
Median	1.5
Range	1–3.7
eGFR (mL/min/1.73 m^2)	
Mean	48
Median	45
Range	15–82
Postoperative hospitalization	**(N = 14)**
Length of stay (days)	
Mean	5.8
Median	5
Range	3–10 months
Day of catheter withdrawal	
Mean	15.5
Median	4.5
Range	3–150 *
Day of drain withdrawal	
Mean	4
Median	3
Range	2–14 months
Complications rated by Clavien-Dindo Score (N = 15)	
0–1	7 (46.6%)
2–3 months	6 (40%)
4	1 (6.66%)
5	1 (6.66%)
Complications noted during postoperative period (N = 15)	
Fever	3
Urosepsis	2
Blood transfusion	5
Atelectasis	3
Surgical site infection	1
Ileus	2
Acute kidney injury	9
Type II MI	1
Sudden cardiac arrest	1
ICU Observation	1

* One patient remained with indwelling catheter until prostatectomy (TUR-P).

4.4. Oncological Outcomes

A period of 12 months was defined as the minimum timeframe for follow-up. This period was characterized by close monitoring; thus, the majority of metastatic or recurrence cases were identified within this timeframe. Although international guidelines indicate that close follow-up has limited evidence for both high- and low-risk disease following radical NU, our institution continues to adhere to this practice, ensuring diligent monitoring [1]. At 12 months, the overall survival and disease-free survival rates were 78.57% and 42.86%, respectively. Of the two patients who received neoadjuvant therapy, one achieved a pathological complete response (pT0) with no evidence of disease (NED) in the 12-month period. Among the six patients who completed adjuvant therapy, two achieved a complete response. Five patients presented with metastatic disease involving the liver, retroperitoneal lymph nodes, lungs, or bones. Among these, three died from the disease within an average of eight months postoperatively. Two patients continued the second-line adjuvant therapy with avelumab. As shown in Table 4, three patients presented with non-urothelial metastatic disease, with recurrence occurring beyond the 12-month follow-up period defined as our study's follow-up timeframe.

Table 4. Twelve-month follow-up.

Total	(N = 14)
Overall survival	**11**
Disease-free survival (UTUC only)	**9**
Cystoscopy follow-up	**9**
Bladder instillation	**2**
Long-term renal failure	
New postoperative onset	6
Progression of chronic kidney injury	3
Dialysis	0
Reoperation	
TURBT	3
NU/BCE resection nest recurrence	0
Imaging follow-up	
PET-CT	11
Metastatic disease	
UC	5
Non-UC	3
Prostate	2
Breast	1
Oncological treatment	
Neoadjuvant	**N = 2**
ddMVAC	1
Gemcitabine + carboplatin	1
Adjuvant	**N = 6**
First line	
Gemcitabine+ cisplatin/carboplatin	3
Pembrolizumab +/− EV	3
Response	
Complete response	2
Partial response	2
Progression	2
Second line (avelumab)	**2**

BCE—bladder cuff excision; ddMVAC—dose-dense methotrexate, vinblastine, doxorubicin, and cisplatin; EV—enfortumab vedotin; NU—nephroureterectomy; UTUC—upper tract urothelial carcinoma.

Bladder Recurrence: Nine patients resumed cystoscopy follow-up; of these, two progressed to metastatic disease. Among the seven non-metastatic patients, three developed bladder recurrence at an average of six months postoperatively, requiring transurethral resection (TURBT) and continued Bacillus Calmette–Guérin (BCG) therapy. One patient refused to undergo BCG instillations.

4.5. Sub-Group Analysis

With regard to Charlson adjusted comorbidity index (CCI): It is important to note that the cohort's population had a median CCI score of 8. To assess whether this technique is suitable for highly morbid patients, we conducted a sub-analysis using a CCI cut-off point of ≥5. A total of 11 out of the 15 patients met this criterion. Among them, two patients died from metastatic disease, one died from cardiac arrest as mentioned, and two patients are still alive, presenting with metastatic UTUC and receiving adjuvant therapy. The overall survival rate in this sub-analysis group was 72.72%, and the disease-free survival rate was 54.54%.

With regard to age: Regarding age, the cohort's median age was 79 years. We conducted a sub-group analysis to assess whether the elderly population would benefit from the procedure, using 80 years as the cut-off. A total of seven patients were 80 years or older. Of them, only one patient died from metastatic disease. The remaining six patients survived with no evidence of disease at the 12-month follow-up. The overall survival rate in this subgroup was 85.71%, with the same rate of disease-free survival.

5. Discussion

Early publications on radical NU involved a combination of laparoscopic nephrectomy and robotic distal ureterectomy with BCE [7]. With technological advancements and increased surgical experience, the robotic approach has become the preferred method for radical NU [8]. However, one of the major drawbacks of RRNU compared to open or laparoscopic approaches is its high cost and time consumption [9]. Despite the minimally invasive nature of the procedure, the prolonged operative time limits its advantages in terms of complication rate [10]. Therefore, optimizing even minor factors to reduce procedure time is essential when performing robotic surgery.

Single-docking robotic NU has been described in the literature, although there is no consensus on the optimal number of ports, their placement, or step-by-step procedural methods. Recent advancements have focused on utilizing the camera-hop technique of the Xi robotic system, which involves intraoperative reconfiguration from the cephalad to caudal direction. Although this approach has been shown to be safe, it has not been universally adopted [11–14].

In our cohort, we employed a relatively under-reported technique for RRNU using only three robotic arm ports and one assistant port: two 8 mm ports for robotic endpoint instruments, one 8 mm port for the camera, and one 12 mm AirSeal assistant port (Figure 1). This minimalist approach allowed for efficient multi-quadrant dissection while minimizing port placement, reducing arm collision, and shortening the overall operative time, thus facilitating a more focused and streamlined surgical process. The intra- and postoperative complications are summarized in Tables 5 and 6, respectively.

The median operative time for our cohort was 133 min, which is significantly lower than the median operative time of 203 min reported by Pathak et al. in their 90-patient cohort using a four-port RRNU technique [13]. Additionally, intraoperative complications in our cohort were minimal, with only two patients requiring blood transfusions, both with controlled bleeding. Importantly, none of the patients required conversion of the surgical approach due to bowel complications. The postoperative major complication rate, defined as Clavien-Dindo grade > III, was 13.33%, which included one death from sudden cardiac arrest and one patient with type II myocardial infarction. These complications should be considered in the context of our patient population, which primarily consisted of patients with a high burden of comorbidities, as reflected by a median CCI of 8 (Table 1). The CCI is designed to preoperatively identify patients at greater risk of intra- and postoperative complications [15]. In our analysis of the subgroup of patients with a CCI $\geq$ 5, we observed a total complication rate of 18%.

The inclusion of octogenarian patients in the surgical management of UTUC has been a frequent focus of previous studies. Large cohorts have demonstrated the benefits of minimally invasive RRNU in elderly populations, emphasizing its low complication rates and relatively high overall survival rates [16–18].

Table 5. Robotic nephroureterectomy—intraoperative variables.

Overall Time (min)	
Mean	162 min
Median	133 min
Range	85–337 min
<150 min	9 (60%)
≥150 min	6 (40%)
Intraoperative additional procedures	
Bladder instillation	2
Time range for intraoperative instillation	112–130 min
Cystoscopy/TURBT	3
Time range for TURBT+NU	209–307 min
Dx URS	1
Time range for Dx URS + cystoscopy + NU	337 min
Lymph nodes dissection	6
Time range for LND + NU	120–253 min
Intraoperative complications	
Bleeding	2 (13.33%)
Blood transfusion	
None	13
1 unit	1
>1 unit	1
EBL	
Mean	200 mL
Median	100 mL
Range	100–1000 mL
Conversion of surgical technique	**0**

Dx URS—diagnostic ureteroscopy; EBL—estimated blood loss; LND—lymph node dissection.

Table 6. Pathology results.

Total	**(N = 15)**
Size	
<4 cm	6
≥4 cm	6
Other	3
Location	
Renal pelvis	6
Proximal ureter	3
Distal ureter	4
Orifice	2
Concurrent bladder	8
Side	
Right	8
Left	7
BCE surgical margins	
R0	15
Clinical TNM	
TaLG	7
TaHG	1
TaLG with 5% HG	1
T1HG	6
Pathological TNM	
T0	3
pT1	4
pT2	2
pT3N0M0	3
pT3N + M+	2
pT4N2M1b	1
Lymph nodes	**(N = 6)**
Positive	2
Negative	4

BCE—bladder cuff excision; HG—high grade; LG—low grade; TNM—tumor, node, distant metastasis staging system.

In our sub-analytical group of patients aged over 80 years, this study corroborates earlier findings, confirming the safety and feasibility of minimally invasive NU. Within this group, we observed a relatively high survival rate of 85.7% and an identical disease remission rate, with a mean follow-up period of 18 months. The complication rate in this subgroup was 14%, comparable to the overall study population.

A review of the literature reveals diverse opinions regarding the factors that most significantly influence surgical outcomes. Wallace et al. reported higher mortality rates among elderly patients; however, their study encompassed 12 different urological procedures rather than focusing solely on NU [19]. In contrast, data from 2,352 patients in the CROES-UTUC registry demonstrated survival benefits associated with radical NU, regardless of age or comorbidities [17].

Our findings suggest that a patient's morbidity profile, as reflected by the CCI, may have a more significant impact on complication rates than age alone [15]. Nonetheless, further prospective studies are necessary to validate these findings.

It is worth noting, however, that the majority of clinical research supports the superiority of radical NU for UTUC, even in the octogenarian population [16,17,20,21]. Multiple clinical trials have compared minimally invasive approaches to open surgery, all indicating the superiority of the minimally invasive approach, particularly robotic surgery [18,21–24]. Unfortunately, one of the drawbacks of the robotic approach, as mentioned, is its time consumption, which may limit its use in the fragile elderly population, further underscoring the advantage of our time-efficient surgical technique [25,26].

While several cohorts have described the use of the camera-hop technique with the da Vinci Xi robotic system for NU, to the best of our knowledge, no study has utilized the three-port single-docking technique described in this report. Studies by Nanigian et al. (2006), Lee et al. (2013), Patel et al. (2015), Pathak et al. (2020), and others have reported various robotic approaches; however, they did not employ this specific configuration [9,13,27,28]. Pathak et al. utilized a four-port technique for RRNU and noted several intraoperative complications, including duodenal injuries, emphasizing the advantage of a reduced-port technique in minimizing the risk of such injuries. Additionally, they suggested that the integration of a movable table could further aid in dissection and prevent arm collisions. Arm collision is another challenge that our three-port technique effectively mitigates, particularly when combined with the Xi arm adjustment switch button [13].

One of the largest studies on RRNU, the ROBUUST cohort, analyzed 1118 patients and reported a median operative time of 212.5 min, along with a postoperative complication rate of 14.1%. While these results provide valuable insights, it is important to note that the ROBUUST study did not standardize robotic system use or surgical techniques, as it included data from multiple centers with varying levels of surgeon expertise. This variability makes direct comparison with our cohort challenging [29]. However, when comparing our results to a more homogeneous group—specifically, the study by Veccia and colleagues published in 2022, which analyzed 148 patients from the ROBUUST cohort who underwent single-stage RRNU with the Xi robotic system—the results were more directly comparable [30]. Their study reported a median operative time of 215.5 min (range: 160.5–290.0), with matched estimated blood loss (EBL) and major complication rates. In contrast, our cohort achieved a median operative time of 133 min, which was considerably shorter, while maintaining a similar complication profile. Although our cohort was small, the results align closely with those of the ROBUUST group in terms of overall complication rates and EBL [29]. Furthermore, our reduced operative time was a notable improvement compared with that of the ROBUUST group, underscoring the time efficiency of our three-port approach. These findings suggest that the three-port technique is not only safe, but also highly time-efficient for performing RRNU (Table 4).

Our study specifically excluded benign cases, focusing solely on malignant UTUC to better evaluate the oncological safety of the three-port single-stage robotic approach. Notably, all patients in our cohort had negative surgical margins, including BCE, and none experienced recurrence in the resection bed during the 12-month follow-up period, even among patients with metastasis (disregarding retroperitoneal lymph nodes). This highlights the oncological efficacy of our technique, which is comparable to that of larger and more complex cohorts.

Our study has several strengths. Uniformity in the surgical technique, patient positioning, trocar placement, intraoperative instruments, and stitches ensured consistency and reliability across all cases. The use of a transperitoneal approach and the Xi robotic program further minimized spillage and optimized procedural time, contributing to the overall efficiency of the technique. However, limitations exist, including the retrospective nature of the study, lack of console time data, and variability in non-robotic procedures such as cystoscopy and Mitomycin C (MMC) instillations. In addition, because the procedure was performed by a single surgeon, the results were subject to performance bias. On the other hand, the experience of a single surgeon enhances the reliability and accuracy of the results, strengthening the feasibility and safety of the three-port single-docking technique.

6. Conclusions

RRNU is a complex procedure that demands a high level of expertise, which can be enhanced through advancements in robotic technology, particularly the upgrade from the X to the Xi robotic platform. Our study demonstrated that the three-port, single-docking NU procedure is both feasible and safe, particularly when the retargeting capabilities of the Xi system are utilized. This cohort achieved the defined tetrafecta for NU, with results comparable to those of the largest published case series using four ports. Notably, the three-port, single-docking technique showed superior performance in terms of overall operative time. To further validate these findings, prospective comparisons between three- and four-port single-docking techniques using the Xi da Vinci program are required. Additionally, the integration of artificial intelligence to optimize camera movement and predict shifts in the surgical field may further improve the efficiency and precision of this approach.

Author Contributions: Conceptualization, Y.Z.; Methodology, Y.Z. and M.H.J.; Software, B.H.; Formal analysis, I.V., R.M. and N.A.; Investigation, E.C. and N.A.; Data curation, Y.Z. and E.M.; Writing—original draft, Y.Z.; Writing—review & editing, Y.Z.; Supervision, N.J.M.; Project administration, N.J.M. All authors have read and agreed to the published version of the manuscript.

Funding: The authors received no financial support for the research, authorship, and publication of this article.

Institutional Review Board Statement: The study was conducted in accordance with the Declaration of Helsinki, and approved by the Institutional Ethics Committee of Soroka University Medical Center (protocol code 0069-24-SOR and date of approval 25 March 2024).

Informed Consent Statement: Patient consent was waived by the Institutional Ethics Committee of Soroka University Medical Center.

Data Availability Statement: The datasets generated and/or analyzed during the current study are available from the corresponding author upon reasonable request.

Conflicts of Interest: The authors declare no conflicts of interest.

Abbreviations

BCE	Bladder cuff excision
BCG	Bacillus Calmette–Guerin
EBL	Estimated blood loss
LND	Lymph node dissection
NU	Nephroureterectomy
MMC	Mitomycin C
POD	Postoperative day
RRNU	Robotic radical nephroureterectomy
TURBT	Transurethral resection of bladder tumor
URS/Dx	URS ureteroscopy/diagnostic ureteroscopy
UTUC	Upper tract urothelial carcinoma

References

1. Rouprêt, M.; Seisen, T.; Birtle, A.J.; Capoun, O.; Compérat, E.M.; Dominguez-Escrig, J.L.; Gürses Andersson, I.; Liedberg, F.; Mariappan, P.; Hugh Mostafid, A.; et al. European Association of Urology Guidelines on Upper Urinary Tract Urothelial Carcinoma: 2023 Update. *Eur. Urol.* **2023**, *84*, 49–64. [CrossRef] [PubMed]
2. Klingler, D.W.; Hemstreet, G.P.; Balaji, K.C. Feasibility of robotic radical nephrectomy—Initial results of single-institution pilot study. *Urology* **2005**, *65*, 1086–1089. [CrossRef] [PubMed]
3. Park, S.K.; Olweny, E.O.; Best, S.L.; Tracy, C.R.; Mir, S.A.; Cadeddu, J.A. Patient-reported body image and cosmesis outcomes following kidney surgery: Comparison of laparoendoscopic single-site, laparoscopic, and open surgery. *Eur. Urol.* **2011**, *60*, 1097–1104. [CrossRef] [PubMed]
4. Pandolfo, S.D.; Cilio, S.; Aveta, A.; Wu, Z.; Cerrato, C.; Napolitano, L.; Lasorsa, F.; Lucarelli, G.; Verze, P.; Siracusano, S.; et al. Upper Tract Urothelial Cancer: Guideline of Guidelines. *Cancers* **2024**, *16*, 1115. [CrossRef]
5. Soria, F.; Pradere, B.; Hurle, R.; D'Andrea, D.; Albisinni, S.; Diamand, R.; Laukhtina, E.; Di Trapani, E.; Aziz, A.; Krajewski, W.; et al. Radical Nephroureterectomy Tetrafecta: A Proposal Reporting Surgical Strategy Quality at Surgery. *Eur. Urol. Open Sci.* **2022**, *42*, 1–8. [CrossRef]
6. Ludwig, W.W.; Gorin, M.A.; Pierorazio, P.M.; Allaf, M.E. Frontiers in robot-assisted retroperitoneal oncological surgery. *Nat. Rev. Urol.* **2017**, *14*, 731–741. [CrossRef]
7. Lai, W.R.; Lee, B.R. Techniques to resect the distal ureter in robotic/laparoscopic nephroureterectomy. *Asian J. Urol.* **2016**, *3*, 120–125. [CrossRef]
8. Saini, S.; Pathak, R.A.; Hemal, A.K. Robotic nephroureterectomy in the management of upper tract urothelial cancer: Inching toward standard of care? *Int. Urol. Nephrol.* **2022**, *54*, 1777–1785. [CrossRef]
9. Patel, M.N.; Aboumohamed, A.; Hemal, A. Does transition from the da Vinci Si ® to Xi robotic platform impact single-docking technique for robot-assisted laparoscopic nephroureterectomy? *BJU Int.* **2015**, *116*, 990–994. [CrossRef]
10. Yip, W.; Assel, M.J.; Wong, N.C.; Tracey, A.T.; Alvim, R.G.; Nogueira, L.; Almassi, N.; Singla, N.; Clinton, T.N.; Sjoberg, D.D.; et al. Changes in the Perioperative Management and Outcomes of Patients with Upper Tract Urothelial Carcinoma Undergoing Radical Nephroureterectomy at Memorial Sloan Kettering Cancer Center: Over 20 Years of Experience. *Urol. Pract.* **2024**, *11*, 356–366. [CrossRef]
11. Darwiche, F.; Swain, S.; Kallingal, G.; Punnen, S.; Manoharan, M.; Parekh, D.J.; Gonzalgo, M.L. Operative technique and early experience for robotic-assisted laparoscopic nephroureterectomy (RALNU) using da Vinci Xi. *SpringerPlus* **2015**, *4*, 298. [CrossRef] [PubMed]
12. Morizane, S.; Yumioka, T.; Iwamoto, H.; Hikita, K.; Honda, M.; Takenaka, A. Initial Experience of Robot-Assisted Laparoscopic Nephroureterectomy in Japan: A Useful Technique Using a Vessel Sealing Device for Securing a Good Surgical Field and Efficient Sealing. *Asian J. Endosc. Surg.* **2022**, *15*, 458–462. [CrossRef]
13. Pathak, R.A.; Dutta, R.; Williams, J.; Hemal, A.K. Robotic radical nephro-ureterectomy for high-risk upper tract urothelial carcinoma: Step-by-step illustrative video of surgical technique. *Urol. Video J.* **2020**, *8*, 100068. [CrossRef]
14. Zargar, H.; Krishnan, J.; Autorino, R.; Akca, O.; Brandao, L.F.; Laydner, H.; Samarasekera, D.; Ko, O.; Haber, G.-P.; Kaouk, J.H.; et al. Robotic Nephroureterectomy: A Simplified Approach Requiring No Patient Repositioning or Robot Redocking. *Eur. Urol.* **2014**, *66*, 769–777. [CrossRef] [PubMed]

15. AlAshqar, A.; Ghazarian, M.; Webster, E.M.; Upadhyay, A.; Azodi, M.; Schwartz, P.E.; Ratner, E.; Altwerger, G. Surgical and oncologic outcomes in surgically treated women 80 years and older with endometrioid endometrial cancer as a function of their comorbidities. *Gynecol. Oncol. Rep.* **2023**, *49*, 101240. [CrossRef]
16. Koterazawa, S.; Kanno, T.; Kobori, G.; Ito, K.; Nakagawa, H.; Takahashi, T.; Takaoka, N.; Somiya, S.; Nagahama, K.; Ito, M.; et al. Clinical outcomes following laparoscopic radical nephroureterectomy in octogenarians. *Int. J. Clin. Oncol.* **2023**, *28*, 155–162. [CrossRef]
17. Teoh, J.Y.C.; Ng, C.F.; Eto, M.; Chiruvella, M.; Capitanio, U.; Esen, T.; Zeng, G.; Lechevallier, E.; Andonian, S.; de la Rosette, J. Radical nephroureterectomy for UTUC conferred survival benefits irrespective of age and comorbidities. *World J. Urol.* **2022**, *40*, 2657–2665. [CrossRef]
18. Trecarten, S.; Bhandari, M.; Abdel-Aziz, A.; Noel, O.; Liss, M.; Dursun, F.; Robert, S.; Mansour, A. Open versus minimally invasive nephroureterectomy in octogenarians: An analysis of surgical approach trends, outcomes and survival analysis with propensity matching. In *Urologic Oncology: Seminars and Original Investigations*; Elsevier: Amsterdam, The Netherlands, 2024; Volume 42.
19. Wallace, B.; Breau, R.H.; Cnossen, S.; Knee, C.; McIsaac, D.; Mallick, R.; Cagiannos, I.; Morash, C.; Lavallée, L.T. Age-stratified perioperative mortality after urological surgeries. *Can. Urol. Assoc. J.* **2018**, *12*, 256. [CrossRef]
20. Upfill-Brown, A.; Lenis, A.T.; Faiena, I.; Salmasi, A.H.; Johnson, D.C.; Pooli, A.; Drakaki, A.; Gollapudi, K.; Blumberg, J.; Pantuck, A.J.; et al. Treatment utilization and overall survival in patients receiving radical nephroureterectomy versus endoscopic management for upper tract urothelial carcinoma: Evaluation of updated treatment guidelines. *World J. Urol.* **2019**, *37*, 1157–1164. [CrossRef]
21. Ye, J.; Wu, Q.; Liao, X.; Zheng, L.; Wei, Q.; Bao, Y. Advanced Age May Not Be an Absolute Contraindication for Radical Nephroureterectomy in Patients with Upper Tract Urothelial Carcinoma: A Single-Center Case Series and a Systematic Review with Meta-Analyses. *J. Clin. Med.* **2023**, *12*, 7273. [CrossRef]
22. Franco, A.; Ditonno, F.; Feng, C.; Manfredi, C.; Sturgis, M.R.; Farooqi, M.; Del Giudice, F.; Coogan, C.; Ferro, M.; Zhang, C.; et al. Minimally Invasive Radical Nephroureterectomy: 5-Year Update of Techniques and Outcomes. *Cancers* **2023**, *15*, 4585. [CrossRef] [PubMed]
23. Lee, H.; Kim, H.J.; Lee, S.E.; Hong, S.K.; Byun, S.S. Comparison of oncological and perioperative outcomes of open, laparoscopic, and robotic nephroureterectomy approaches in patients with non-metastatic upper-tract urothelial carcinoma. *PLoS ONE* **2019**, *14*, 401. [CrossRef] [PubMed]
24. Rajan, K.; Khalifa, A.; Geraghty, R.; Parmar, K.; KandaSwamy, G.; Gómez Rivas, J.; Somani, B.; Rai, B.P. Oncological Efficacy of Robotic Nephroureterectomy vs. Open and Laparoscopic Nephroureterectomy for Suspected Non-Metastatic UTUC—A Systematic Review and Meta-Analysis. *Cancers* **2023**, *15*, 4926. [CrossRef] [PubMed]
25. Maynou, L.; McGuire, A.; Serra-Sastre, V. Efficiency and Productivity Gains of Robotic Surgery: The Case of the English National Health Service. *SSRN Electron. J.* **2023**, *33*, 820. [CrossRef]
26. Reddy, K.; Gharde, P.; Tayade, H.; Patil, M.; Reddy, L.S.; Surya, D. Advancements in Robotic Surgery: A Comprehensive Overview of Current Utilizations and Upcoming Frontiers. *Cureus* **2023**, *15*, e50415. [CrossRef]
27. Lee, Z.; Cadillo-Chavez, R.; Lee, D.I.; Llukani, E.; Eun, D. The Technique of Single Stage Pure Robotic Nephroureterectomy. *J. Endourol.* **2013**, *27*, 189–195. [CrossRef]
28. Nanigian, D.K.; Smith, W.; Ellison, L.M. Robot-Assisted Laparoscopic Nephroureterectomy. *J. Endourol.* **2006**, *20*, 463–466. [CrossRef]
29. Ditonno, F.; Franco, A.; Wu, Z.; Wang, L.; Abdollah, F.; Simone, G.; Correa, A.F.; Ferro, M.; Perdonà, S.; Amparore, D.; et al. Robot-assisted nephroureterectomy: Surgical and mid-term oncological outcomes in over 1100 patients (ROBUUST 2.0 collaborative group). *BJU Int.* **2024**, *134*, 967–975. [CrossRef]
30. Veccia, A.; Carbonara, U.; Derweesh, I.; Mehrazin, R.; Porter, J.; Abdollah, F.; Mazzone, E.; Sundaram, C.P.; Gonzalgo, M.; Mastroianni, R.; et al. Single-stage Xi® robotic radical nephroureterectomy for upper tract urothelial carcinoma: Surgical technique and outcomes. *Minerva Urol. Nephrol.* **2022**, *74*, 233–241. [CrossRef]

cancers

MDPI

rticle

Robot-Assisted Radical Nephroureterectomy: A Safe and Effective Option for Upper Tract Urothelial Carcinoma, Especially for Novice Surgeons

Chia-Lun Chang [1,2], Chung-You Tsai [3,4], Pai-Yu Cheng [3,5], Wen-Jeng Wu [6,7,8] and Yao-Chou Tsai [1,2,*]

1 Division of Urology, Department of Surgery, Taipei Tzu Chi Hospital, The Buddhist Medical Foundation, New Taipei 231405, Taiwan; mr.tony1990@gmail.com
2 School of Medicine, Buddhist Tzu Chi University, Hualien 97004, Taiwan
3 Division of Urology, Department of Surgery, Far Eastern Memorial Hospital, New Taipei 220216, Taiwan; pgtsai@gmail.com (C.-Y.T.); zack00693@gmail.com (P.-Y.C.)
4 Department of Electrical Engineering, Yuan-Ze University, Chung-Li 32003, Taiwan
5 Department of Biomedical Engineering, National Taiwan University, Taipei 10617, Taiwan
6 Department of Urology, Kaohsiung Medical University Hospital, Kaohsiung 80756, Taiwan; wejewu@kmu.edu.tw
7 Department of Urology, School of Medicine, College of Medicine, Kaohsiung Medical University, Kaohsiung 80708, Taiwan
8 Graduate Institute of Clinical Medicine, College of Medicine, Kaohsiung Medical University, Kaohsiung 80708, Taiwan
* Correspondence: tsai1970523@yahoo.com.tw; Tel.: +886-2-66289779 (ext. 2241)

Simple Summary: This study compared robotic (RARNU) and laparoscopic (LRNU) surgery for treating upper tract urothelial carcinoma (UTUC). Researchers analyzed data from over 2037 Taiwanese patients and found that both approaches had similar outcomes in terms of complications, cancer recurrence, and survival rates. While both methods were effective, the study suggests that robotic surgery might be easier for surgeons to adopt, especially those with less experience in laparoscopic techniques.

Abstract: Background: Radical nephroureterectomy (RNU) is the standard treatment for upper tract urothelial carcinoma (UTUC). Minimally invasive techniques like robotic (RARNU) and laparoscopic (LRNU) RNU offer potential benefits over open surgery, but their comparative oncologic outcomes are debated. Methods: This retrospective, multicenter study analyzed 2037 Taiwanese patients undergoing RNU between 2010 and 2022. Missing data was addressed using multiple imputations. Overlap weighting was applied to balance patient characteristics between the RARNU and LRNU groups. Survival outcomes were compared using Kaplan-Meier analysis and Cox regression. Results: After excluding the missing data, 405 patients underwent RARNU, and 1262 underwent LRNU. After adjusting for baseline differences, both groups showed comparable rates of surgical complications, residual tumor, UTUC-related mortality, and disease recurrence. The median follow-up was similar (52.4 vs. 51.6 months, $p = 0.91$). Using Kaplan-Meier survival curve analysis, overall survival, cancer-specific survival, and disease-free survival were similar between the two groups. Conclusions: This study shows that RARNU for UTUC has comparable oncological and perioperative outcomes to pure LRNU. RARNU may be easier for surgeons to adopt, particularly those with limited laparoscopic experience.

Keywords: robotic; laparoscopic; nephroureterectomy; upper urinary tract urothelial cancer

1. Introduction

Upper tract urothelial carcinoma (UTUC) is rare, making up 5–10% of urothelial cancers in the West, but has a significantly higher incidence (20–30%) in Taiwan [1–5]. Unlike other regions, Taiwan also shows a higher prevalence of UTUC among women, suggesting a unique cancer behavior [6,7]. Radical nephroureterectomy (RNU) with bladder cuff excision is the standard treatment for UTUC [8]. Traditionally performed using an open approach, the rise of minimally invasive techniques has transformed the surgical landscape by offering advantages such as smaller incisions, better cosmetic results, reduced bleeding, and faster postoperative recovery [9]. The use of laparoscopic and robot-assisted RNU increased from 36% to 54% between 2004 and 2013 [10]. Several studies have shown that LRNU and RARNU offer reduced perioperative morbidity and comparable oncological control compared to the open approach [11–13]. However, the potential for incomplete tumor resection, increased tumor recurrence, and long-term oncological outcomes associated with minimally invasive approaches—including LRNU and RARNU—remain debated, with mixed results in the literature [14–17]. Moreover, many previous studies have analyzed small cohorts commonly enrolled using the hand-assisted approach and often failed to assess oncological outcomes comprehensively [10,18,19]. In contrast to the hand-assisted laparoscopic approach, pure LRNU presents a steeper learning curve and poses significant challenges, particularly in managing the bladder cuff. These conflicting findings underscore the need for more rigorous and comprehensive analyses to better understand the true benefits and limitations of pure LRNU and RARNU in the treatment of UTUC. This study aims to comprehensively compare the safety, efficacy, and impact of pure LRNU and RARNU for UTUC during the learning curve in a multi-institutional Taiwanese cohort. The findings will inform clinical decision-making and optimize surgical management strategies for patients with UTUC.

2. Materials and Methods

2.1. Study Population

The Taiwan UTUC Collaboration Group Database compiled clinical and pathological data of UTUC patients from 21 hospitals across Taiwan. This study retrospectively analyzed data from patients who underwent RARNU or LRNU, including laparoendoscopic single-site (LESS) RNU, between 2010 and 2022. Exclusion criteria included clinical evidence of metastatic disease at the time of surgery, a prior history of cystectomy for bladder cancer, hand-assisted LRNU, and variant UTUC subtypes. Out of 2037 patients assessed for eligibility, 1667 were included in the final analysis (Figure 1 flow diagram). All the participants underwent RNU with bladder cuff excision. Lymph node dissection was performed only for those with suspected lymph node involvement, with the extent determined by the surgeon. Decisions regarding neoadjuvant or adjuvant chemotherapy were based on the patient's clinical staging and overall condition, as decided by the treating physician and patient. This retrospective analysis was approved by the Institutional Review Board of Taipei Tzu Chi Hospital (No. 06-X34-105).

2.2. Definitions and Endpoints

Pathological staging was based on the 2010 TNM (tumor, lymph node, metastasis) system, and tumor grading followed the 2004 WHO/International Society of Urologic Pathology classification. Postoperative complications were classified using the Clavien–Dindo system. Recurrence was confirmed by cross-sectional imaging and/or pathological examination, including local recurrence at the tumor bed, lymph nodes, or distant sites. Disease-free survival (DFS) was defined as the time from surgery to the first recurrence, while overall survival (OS) was defined as the time from surgery to death from any cause.

The cause of death was determined mainly from death certificates, with medical records reviewed when unclear. The study's endpoints were the comparison of oncological outcomes and safety between RARNU and LRNU, specifically focusing on overall survival (OS), cancer-specific survival (CSS), and disease-free survival (DFS).

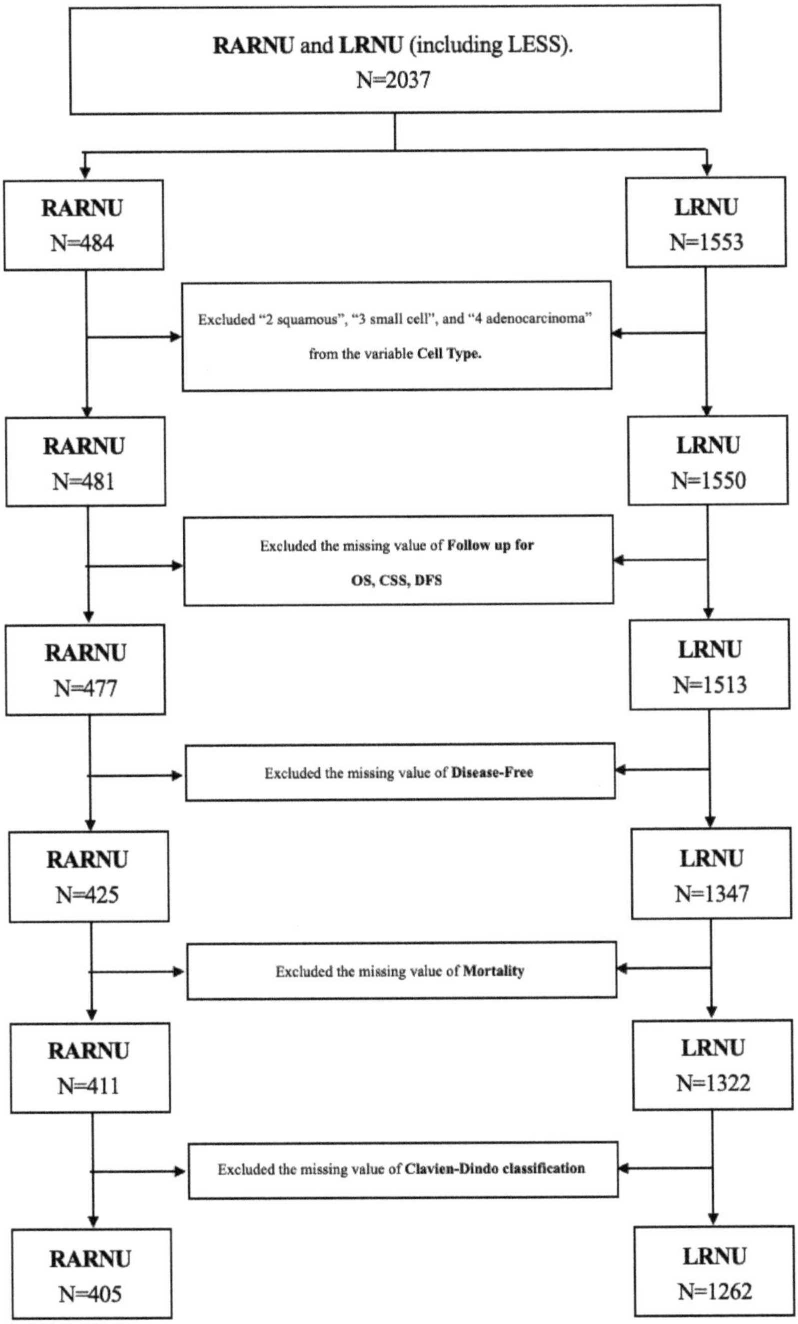

Figure 1. Study flow diagram.

2.3. Follow-Up Protocols

Patients were generally evaluated every 3–6 months through a medical history review, physical examination, urine cytology, renal ultrasound, and cystoscopy. Abdominal computed tomography (CT) or magnetic resonance imaging (MRI) was performed every 6–12 months to monitor for recurrence. If clinically indicated, chest CT or a bone scan was conducted to check for distant metastasis.

2.4. Statistical Analysis

Differences between the RARNU and LRNU (including LESS) groups were assessed using standardized mean differences for both categorical and continuous variables. Approximately 4% of the data had missing values across some variables. We addressed these missing values using multiple imputations by chained equations (MICE), a commonly applied method in literature. To assess the performance of MICE in our context, we simulated a dataset with missing values similar to those observed. We first created a complete dataset by removing all rows containing missing values from the original data, which consisted of 1028 patients and 30 variables. From this complete dataset, we randomly deleted 5000 values from the variables that originally had missing data to construct a testing dataset with simulated missingness. The accuracy of the MICE imputations, averaged over 30 trials, was 0.72 [20] reported that acceptable accuracy in machine learning models typically ranges from 0.7 to 0.9; our results indicate that MICE performed adequately in this scenario.

To balance the two groups, we applied overlap weighting to adjust for baseline differences. Overlap weighting is a propensity score (PS) matching method that has several advantages over other PS matching methods, including: (1) It creates an exact balance on the mean of every measured covariate when the PS is estimated by logistic regression. This is particularly important for reducing bias, as it ensures that the treatment and control groups are comparable in all the measured confounders. (2) It can be used even when there are no overlaps between the treatment and control groups on the PS distribution, which is common in a retrospective setting. (3) It does not require trimming of case numbers. (4) Overlap weighting has been shown to minimize the variance of the weighted estimator of the treatment effect among all the balancing weights, including inverse probability of treatment weighting (IPTW). This means that overlap weighting is more efficient than other PS matching methods in terms of precision [21,22]. After the overlap weighting, the love plot revealed a balanced standardized mean difference across LRNU vs. RARNU groups among all variables with the overlap technique (Supplementary Figure S1: Love Plot). In addition, the performance of overlap weighting was clearly better than the inverse probability treatment weighting technique.

For the survival analyses, we prioritized variable selection using the Akaike Information Criterion (AIC) and Lasso regression to identify the most relevant variables. The Kaplan-Meier estimator, combined with Cox regression modeling, was then used to generate and visualize the overall, cancer-specific, and disease-free survival curves.

3. Results

3.1. Baseline Characteristics

A total of 2037 patients who underwent minimally invasive radical nephroureterectomy (RNU) across 21 centers in Taiwan were analyzed. After excluding missing values and imputing missing data using multiple imputations by chained equations (MICE), 405 patients had robot-assisted RNU (RARNU) and 1262 had pure laparoscopic RNU (LRNU) for final analysis (Table 1).

Table 1. Comparison of baseline patient characteristics, tumor characteristics, pathological findings, postoperative complications, and treatment outcomes in UTUC patients undergoing robot-assisted or laparoscopic radical nephroureterectomy after multiple imputation with chained equations.

		RARNU	LRNU	*p*	SMD
N		405	1262		
	NU	394	1257		
	Segmental	11	5		
ECOG (%)	0	211 (52.1)	631 (50.0)	0.217	0.153
	1	172 (42.5)	521 (41.3)		
	2	20 (4.9)	89 (7.1)		
	3	2 (0.5)	16 (1.3)		
	4	0 (0.0)	5 (0.4)		
Sex (%)	Male	172 (42.5)	520 (41.2)	0.695	0.026
	Female	233 (57.5)	742 (58.8)		
Age (mean (SD))		69.25 (10.26)	68.15 (10.51)	0.066 *	0.106
BMI (%)	Normal	241 (59.5)	776 (61.5)	0.513	0.041
	Overweight	164 (40.5)	486 (38.5)		
Cell Type (%)	Urothelial	346 (85.4)	1124 (89.1)	0.126	0.112
	UC with variants	55 (13.6)	131 (10.4)		
	Others	4 (1.0)	7 (0.6)		
Side (%)	Left	209 (51.6)	643 (51.0)	0.948	0.019
	Right	189 (46.7)	599 (47.5)		
	Both	7 (1.7)	20 (1.6)		
Location (%)	Non-Visible	1 (0.2)	1 (0.1)	0.645	0.086
	Renal Pelvis	163 (40.2)	546 (43.3)		
	Ureter	142 (35.1)	402 (31.9)		
	Bladder Cuff	1 (0.2)	2 (0.2)		
	Multiple	98 (24.2)	311 (24.6)		
Multiple (%)	No	262 (64.7)	825 (65.4)	0.849	0.014
	Yes	143 (35.3)	437 (34.6)		
Size (%)	<2 cm	131 (32.3)	416 (33.0)	0.865	0.013
	≥2 cm	274 (67.7)	846 (67.0)		
Pathological Stage (%)	Stage 0a/0is	64 (15.8)	204 (16.2)	0.167	0.14
	Stage I	104 (25.7)	359 (28.4)		
	Stage II	70 (17.3)	238 (18.9)		
	Stage III	125 (30.9)	375 (29.7)		
	Stage IV	42 (10.4)	86 (6.8)		
Grade (%)	Low Grade	43 (10.6)	122 (9.7)	0.001 **	0.237
	High Grade	351 (86.7)	1039 (82.3)		
	Not Available	11 (2.7)	101 (8.0)		
Bladder Cancer (%)	No	316 (78.0)	936 (74.2)	0.268	0.094
	Previous History of Bladder UC	24 (5.9)	96 (7.6)		
	Concurrent Bladder UC	65 (16.0)	230 (18.2)		
CIS (%)	No	280 (69.1)	919 (72.8)	0.17	0.081
	Yes	125 (30.9)	343 (27.2)		
LVI (%)	No	326 (80.5)	1051 (83.3)	0.226	0.072
	Yes	79 (19.5)	211 (16.7)		
Surgical Margin (%)	Free	384 (94.8)	1226 (97.1)	0.037 *	0.119
	Positive	21 (5.2)	36 (2.9)		
Pre-operation Hydronephrosis (%)	No	230 (56.8)	660 (52.3)	0.129	0.09
	Yes	175 (43.2)	602 (47.7)		

Table 1. *Cont.*

		RARNU	LRNU	*p*	SMD
Tumor Necrosis (%)	No	352 (86.9)	1079 (85.5)	0.53	0.041
	Yes	53 (13.1)	183 (14.5)		
Chemotherapy Type (%)	No	275 (67.9)	907 (71.9)	0.062 *	0.128
	Peri-OP Adjuvant	99 (24.4)	295 (23.4)		
	Salvage/Palliative	31 (7.7)	60 (4.8)		
Bladder Cuff Resection (%)	Not Perform BCR	11 (2.7)	42 (3.3)	<0.001 ***	2.402
	Open Incision	81 (20.0)	879 (69.7)		
	Residual Bladder Cuff (%)	14 (17.3)	166 (18.9)		
	Transurethral Incision	9 (2.2)	52 (4.1)		
	Laparoscopy	7 (1.7)	284 (22.5)		
	Residual Bladder Cuff (%)		46 (16.2)		
	Robot-Assisted	297 (73.3)	5 (0.4)		
	Residual Bladder Cuff (%)	42 (14.1)			
Post-Operation Intravesical C/T Instillation (%)	No	335 (82.7)	1200 (95.1)	<0.001 ***	0.402
	Intravesical Therapy	70 (17.3)	62 (4.9)		

RARNU: robot-assisted radical nephroureterectomy, LRNU: laparoscopic radical nephroureterectomy, SMD: standardized mean difference, NU: nephroureterectomy, UC: urothelial carcinoma, CIS: carcinoma in situ, LVI: lymphovascular invasion, C/T: chemotherapy, *p*: <0.1 *, <0.01 **, <0.001 ***.

Before overlap weighting, the baseline characteristics were comparable among most variables, except for surgical margin status, bladder cuff resection methods, and postoperative intravesical chemotherapy status. The RARNU group was associated with a higher rate of high-grade histology and positive surgical margins (5.2% vs. 2.9%, $p = 0.037$). Additionally, nearly 75% of bladder cuffs in the RARNU group were managed endoscopically, compared to only 23% in the LRNU group. Intravesical chemotherapy after RNU was administered to a limited number of patients in both groups (17.3% vs. 4.9%, $p < 0.001$).

3.2. Surgical Outcomes

After overlap weighting, the standardized mean differences were well-balanced across groups for all baseline characteristics (Supplementary Figure S1). The mean age in the RARNU group was 69.25 ± 10.26 years and 68.15 ± 10.51 years in the LRNU group (Table 1).

The outcome variables derived after overlap weighting revealed comparable rates of Clavien-Dindo surgical complications, rate of residual bladder cuff, UTUC-related mortality, and disease recurrence between the two groups, with comparable median follow-up periods (52.4 ± 33.4 vs. 51.6 ± 37.8 months, $p = 0.91$) (Table 2). The Kaplan–Meier survival curve analysis demonstrated similar OS, CSS, and DFS between the two groups (Figure 2).

Table 2. Outcome variable comparisons between robot-assisted or laparoscopic radical nephroureterectomy groups before and after overlap weighting.

		Overlap				Unweighted			
		RARNU	LRNU	*p*	SMD	RARNU	LRNU	*p*	SMD
Clavien-Dindo Classification (%)	No Complication	468.6 (56.3)	541.5 (65.0)	0.122	0.245	259 (64.0)	861 (68.2)	0.079 *	0.180
	Grade I	154.7 (18.6)	105.3 (12.6)			66 (16.3)	148 (11.7)		
	Grade II	194.4 (23.3)	160.5 (19.3)			71 (17.5)	205 (16.2)		
	Grade III	14.7 (1.8)	18.2 (2.2)			6 (1.5)	31 (2.4)		
	Grade IV	0.3 (0.0)	7.3 (0.9)			2 (0.5)	16 (1.3)		
	Grade V	0.2 (0.0)	0.1 (0.0)			1 (0.2)	1 (0.1)		

Table 2. *Cont.*

		Overlap				Unweighted			
		RARNU	LRNU	*p*	SMD	RARNU	LRNU	*p*	SMD
Residual Bladder Cuff (%)	No Yes	656.1 (78.8) 176.9 (21.2)	652.7 (78.4) 180.3 (21.6)	0.921	0.010	339 (83.7) 66 (16.3)	1020 (80.8) 242 (19.2)	0.22	0.075
Overall Mortality (%) (Within 5 years)	No Yes	575.5 (69.1) 257.5 (30.9)	487.2 (58.5) 345.8 (41.5)	0.034 *	0.222	285 (70.4) 120 (29.6)	747 (59.2) 515 (40.8)	<0.001 ***	0.236
UTUC Mortality (%) (Within 5 years)	No Yes	687.8 (82.6) 145.2 (17.4)	696.1 (83.6) 136.9 (16.4)	0.793	0.027	344 (84.9) 61 (15.1)	1102 (87.3) 160 (12.7)	0.252	0.069
Disease-Free (%)	No Yes	176.1 (21.1) 656.9 (78.9)	183.4 (22.0) 649.6 (78.0)	0.834	0.021	98 (24.2) 307 (75.8)	244 (19.3) 1018 (80.7)	0.042 *	0.118
Bladder Recurrence (%)	No Yes	616.4 (74.0) 216.6 (26.0)	615.5 (73.9) 217.5 (26.1)	0.981	0.002	308 (76.0) 97 (24.0)	921 (73.0) 341 (27.0)	0.247	0.07
Follow-Up OS/CSS (Mean(SD))		52.03 (33.43)	51.65 (37.79)	0.913	0.011	44.45 (30.64)	52.51 (38.88)	<0.001 ***	0.23

RARNU: robot-assisted radical nephroureterectomy, LRNU: laparoscopic radical nephroureterectomy, SMD: standardized mean difference, UTUC: upper tract urothelial carcinoma, OS: overall survival, CSS: cancer-specific survival, *p*: <0.1 *, <0.001 ***.

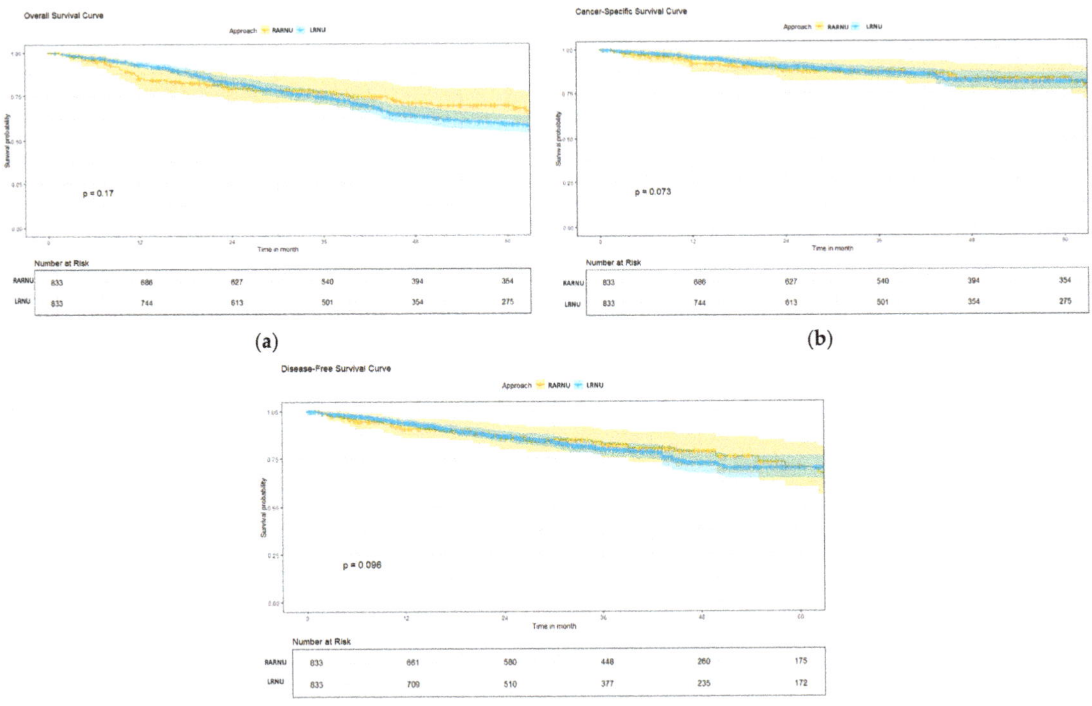

Figure 2. Survival analysis of UTUC patients with robot-assisted or laparoscopic radical nephroureterectomy using Kaplan-Meier method (**a**) 5-year overall survival, (**b**) 5-year cancer-specific survival, and (**c**) 5-year disease-free survival.

3.3. Survival Prediction Model

Multivariate survival analysis revealed comparable OS, CSS, and DFS between the two groups (Table 3). Independent risk factors for OS included higher ECOG, higher age, multiplicity, advanced pathological stage, and positive surgical margin. Independent risk factors for CSS included higher age, advanced pathological stage, multiplicity, tumor > 2 cm, LVI, and positive surgical margin. Independent risk factors for DFS included higher age, multiplicity, advanced pathological stage, concurrent bladder urothelial carcinoma (UC), lymphovascular invasion (LVI), positive surgical margin, and hydronephrosis.

Table 3. Multivariable Cox regression analyses assessing the association of each variable with overall survival, cancer-specific survival, and disease-free survival in UTUC patients undergoing robot-assisted or laparoscopic radical nephroureterectomy.

		OS		CSS		DFS	
		HR (95%CI)	*p*	**HR (95%CI)**	*p*	**HR (95%CI)**	*p*
Approach	RARNU	1		1		1	
	LRNU	1.21 (0.85, 1.71)	0.298	0.80 (0.49, 1.30)	0.362	0.80 (0.63, 1.02)	0.071 *
ECOG	0	1				1	
	1	1.22 (1.03, 1.46)	0.024 *			1.33 (1.06, 1.68)	0.015 *
	2	1.82 (1.38, 2.41)	<0.001 ***			1.29 (0.84, 1.99)	0.25
	3	2.02 (1.20, 3.38)	0.008 **			1.74 (0.54, 5.57)	0.352
	4	1.53 (0.56, 4.19)	0.406			2.06 (0.28,14.92)	0.476
Sex	Male	1		1			
	Female	0.80 (0.68, 0.95)	0.009 **	0.70 (0.53, 0.92)	0.010 *		
Age	Mean	1.03 (1.02, 1.04)	<0.001 ***	1.04 (1.02, 1.05)	<0.001 ***	1.03 (1.01, 1.04)	<0.001 ***
BMI	Normal	1					
	Overweight	0.79 (0.67, 0.94)	0.007 **				
Multiple	No	1		1		1	
	Yes	1.22 (1.04, 1.45)	0.017 *	1.65 (1.26, 2.16)	<0.001 ***	1.26 (1.00, 1.58)	0.049 *
Size	<2 cm			1		1	
	≥2 cm			1.50 (1.02, 2.19)	0.038 *	1.28 (0.96, 1.71)	0.087 *
Pathological Stage	Stage 0a/0is	1		1		1	
	Stage I	1.34 (0.98, 1.83)	0.067 *	2.32 (0.96, 5.63)	0.062 *	1.31 (0.76, 2.25)	0.327
	Stage II	1.35 (0.96, 1.90)	0.088 *	3.58 (1.48, 8.66)	0.005 **	1.84 (1.06, 3.17)	0.030 *
	Stage III	2.04 (1.47, 2.84)	<0.001 ***	5.25 (2.22, 12.42)	<0.001 ***	3.32 (1.97, 5.60)	<0.001 ***
	Stage IV	5.06 (3.35, 7.64)	<0.001 ***	13.81 (5.55, 34.36)	<0.001 ***	8.31 (4.62,14.93)	<0.001 ***

Table 3. *Cont.*

		OS		CSS		DFS	
		HR (95%CI)	*p*	HR (95%CI)	*p*	HR (95%CI)	*p*
Grade	Low Grade	1					
	High Grade	1.58 (1.08, 2.32)	0.019 *				
	Not Available	3.13 (2.03, 4.83)	<0.001 ***				
Bladder Cancer	No	1				1	
	Previous History of Bladder UC	0.99 (0.72, 1.37)	0.957			1.36 (0.85, 2.17)	0.204
	Concurrent Bladder UC	1.23 (1.01, 1.51)	0.043 *			1.36 (1.02, 1.80)	0.034 *
CIS	No	1				1	
	Yes	0.81 (0.67, 0.98)	0.026 *			0.75 (0.59, 0.96)	0.023 *
LVI	No	1		1		1	
	Yes	1.19 (0.97, 1.47)	0.096 *	1.42 (1.04, 1.93)	0.025 *	1.37 (1.06, 1.77)	0.015 *
Surgical Margin	Free	1		1		1	
	Positive	1.64 (1.14, 2.35)	0.007 **	1.67 (1.05, 2.65)	0.029 *	1.70 (1.16, 2.47)	0.006 **
Pre-operation Hy-dronephrosis	No					1	
	Yes					0.78 (0.62, 0.99)	0.039 *
Bladder Cuff Resection	Not Perform BCR	1		1			
	Open Incision	0.52 (0.34, 0.79)	0.002 **	0.57 (0.28, 1.19)	0.137		
	Transurethral Incision	0.31 (0.17, 0.56)	<0.001 ***	0.53 (0.21, 1.34)	0.181		
	Laparoscopy	0.39 (0.25, 0.61)	<0.001 ***	0.50 (0.23, 1.07)	0.075 *		
	Robot-Assisted	0.48 (0.28, 0.83)	0.009 **	0.44 (0.19, 1.03)	0.058 *		
Residual Bladder Cuff	No	1		1		1	
	Yes	0.54 (0.42, 0.70)	<0.001 ***	0.55 (0.36, 0.82)	0.004 **	0.76 (0.58, 1.01)	0.058 *

RARNU: robot-assisted radical nephroureterectomy, LRNU: laparoscopic radical nephroureterectomy, HR: hazard ratio, CI: confidence interval, OS: overall survival, CSS: cancer-specific survival, DFS: disease-free survival, UC: urothelial carcinoma, CIS: carcinoma in situ, LVI: lymphovascular invasion, *p*: <0.1 *, <0.01 **, <0.001 ***.

3.4. Surgeon Experience

In our sub-analysis, the median surgical loads per doctor were three for the RARNU group and four for the LRNU group. The average surgical loads per doctor were 8.21 for the RARNU group and 8.52 for the laparoscopic surgery LRNU group. Additionally, according to the case load plot, nearly half (25/56) of robotic surgeons had no or minimal experience (less than 10 cases in LRNU). (Supplementary Figure S2).

4. Discussion

Robot-assisted radical nephroureterectomy (RARNU) offers several advantages over open surgery, including smaller incisions, improved cosmetic outcomes, reduced blood loss, and faster postoperative recovery [23]. While laparoscopic radical nephroureterectomy (LRNU) shares these benefits, its steep learning curve has hindered widespread adoption of minimally invasive approaches in renal surgery [24]. The introduction of robotic platforms has facilitated the transition from open to minimally invasive surgery, making endoscopic urological procedures more accessible to patients and surgeons alike [25,26]. Our multicenter study represents one of the largest cohort analyses comparing surgical and oncological outcomes for upper tract urothelial carcinoma (UTUC) patients undergoing robotic and pure laparoscopic RNU. We found that RARNU was associated with comparable hospital stays, surgical complications, and survival outcomes compared to pure LRNU. These findings suggest that RARNU is a safe and effective surgical option for UTUC and may provide a more accessible pathway for open surgeons to adopt minimally invasive techniques.

Robotic surgical systems have significantly advanced minimally invasive surgery, empowering surgeons to perform complex procedures endoscopically with greater precision, dexterity, and control [9,27]. Radical prostatectomy (RP), one of the most intricate endoscopic procedures in urology, exemplifies this revolution. In the United States, a national survey between 1998 and 2011 demonstrated a rapid expansion of minimally invasive RP, driven by the widespread adoption of da Vinci Surgical Systems [28]. Notably, during this period, laparoscopic RP declined to less than 10% of all RP procedures, highlighting the versatility and ease of adaptation of the robotic platform for open-incision surgeons. Although the da Vinci Surgical System received FDA approval in Taiwan in 2004, the first case of RARNU in the country was performed in 2011, marking the start of the learning curve for RARNU in this cohort study. According to the case load plot, approximately half of the robotic surgeons had experience with fewer than 10 LRNU cases. Although a significant proportion of surgeons in the RARNU group had no experience or were in their early learning curve, both groups had comparable surgical and oncological outcomes. Therefore, the RARNU approach is a versatile and user-friendly procedure, particularly for young and novice surgeons, with similar surgical outcomes to its pure laparoscopic counterpart.

Bladder cuff resection is one of the critical components of radical nephroureterectomy, particularly for tumors located in the lower ureter or bladder cuff. Pure endoscopic management of the bladder cuff offers several advantages, including smaller incisions, reduced blood loss, faster recovery, and potentially decreased risks of open wound-related complications [29]. However, laparoscopic techniques, while minimally invasive, have been associated with a higher incidence of positive surgical margins and local recurrence in some smaller retrospective studies [30,31]. Additionally, the technical challenges of intracorporeal suturing can limit the widespread adoption of laparoscopic approaches, especially for open-incision surgeons. In contrast, RARNU provides a more versatile and accessible platform for bladder cuff resection. The 3D magnified view and enhanced dexterity afforded by robotic technology allow for precise dissection and suturing, even in complex cases. Our multicenter study demonstrated that RARNU facilitated endoscopic bladder cuff resection in over 70% of cases, compared to only 25% in the laparoscopic group. Though most bladder cuffs were managed endoscopically in the RARNU group during the learning curve, the RARNU group actually had a similar bladder cuff residual rate (21.7 vs. 21.4%, $p = 0.95$) and bladder recurrence rate (26.0 vs. 26.1%, $p = 0.98$) as the LRNU group (Table 2). Moreover, the current study and other large-scale studies have all shown that RARNU does not increase the risk of positive surgical margins or disease recurrence [11,17,32]. Hence, robot-assisted surgery offers a safe, effective, and more versatile endoscopic approach to bladder cuff resection during radical nephroureterectomy.

The results in Table 3 also demonstrated that there was no statistically significant difference between the RARNU and LRNU groups in terms of OS, CSS, or DFS in this multivariable model. This finding is central to our comparison, suggesting that after accounting for other factors, the surgical approach itself does not independently impact long-term oncological outcomes within our study cohort. The absence of a significant difference between the groups in this analysis supports our findings regarding the comparable long-term effectiveness of both techniques. By combining the benefits of minimally invasive surgery with enhanced surgical precision, the robotic platform provides a valuable tool to optimize patient outcomes and minimize complications in bladder cuff resection.

Hand-assisted laparoscopic nephroureterectomy (HALRNU) can help overcome the learning curve associated with the pure laparoscopic approach for upper tract urothelial carcinoma (UTUC). Historical comparative cohorts for robotic versus laparoscopic RNU commonly enrolled cases using the hand-assisted approach for LRNU [33]. While HALRNU might shorten operative times due to hand assistance for blunt dissection and tactile feedback, this advantage does not significantly impact overall survival, cancer-specific mortality, or extra-vesical recurrence rates. However, HALRNU may increase the risk of intravesical recurrence and a higher rate of disease recurrence following RNU [33,34]. This could be due to the increased possibility of genitourinary tract manipulation during hand-assisted surgery, thus increasing the chance of tumor dissemination to the urinary bladder or lymphatic tracts, leading to disease recurrence. In our cohort analysis, RARNU not only performed as well as pure LRNU but also maintained the treatment quality of pure LRNU during the learning phase. Therefore, RARNU should be recommended as the treatment of choice for novice surgeons treating UTUC.

While RARNU offers several advantages over LRNU, such as a more user-friendly surgical platform for novice surgeons, improved surgeon ergonomics, and potentially easier endoscopic bladder cuff management, it is not without its drawbacks. Firstly, RARNU typically requires a longer operative time compared to LRNU [35]. Secondly, the use of robotic systems often results in higher surgical costs. These increased costs stem from the significant expense of acquiring and maintaining the robotic equipment [35,36]. Finally, not all medical centers have access to robotic surgical systems, which can limit the availability of RARNU for patients [37]. Therefore, the choice between RARNU and LRNU should be made on a case-by-case basis, through careful discussion between the patient and their urologist. This discussion should consider several factors, including surgeon proficiency with both techniques, availability of robotic platforms, patient affordability, and hospital resources.

Our study should be addressed with some limitations. Being a retrospective study, it inherently carries the potential for bias and confounding variables. The multicenter nature of the study, involving different surgeons, adds to the heterogeneous nature of the data. Different surgeons with varying levels of experience and differing surgical methods may have influenced the results. However, the study was strengthened by its real-world data analysis with a large sample size and comprehensive correction for confounding covariates.

5. Conclusions

This study demonstrates that RARNU is a safe and effective surgical option for the treatment of UTUC. Our findings show that RARNU is associated with comparable oncological and perioperative outcomes to pure laparoscopic radical nephroureterectomy, including similar rates of complications, recurrence, and survival. Importantly, RARNU may provide a more user-friendly and accessible pathway for surgeons, particularly those with limited laparoscopic experience, to adopt minimally invasive techniques.

Supplementary Materials: The following supporting information can be downloaded at: https://www.mdpi.com/article/10.3390/cancers17091394/s1, Figure S1: Love plot of the absolute standardized difference for each covariate in the original and weighted data: IPTW: inverse probability treatment weighting; overlap: overlap weighting; Figure S2: Case load plot illustrating the number of robotic-assisted and laparoscopic radical nephroureterectomy procedures performed by each surgeon.

Author Contributions: Y.-C.T., C.-Y.T., P.-Y.C. and W.-J.W. conceptualized and designed the study, and performed data collection and data analysis; C.-L.C. drafted the original manuscript. C.-L.C. and Y.-C.T. coordinated and supervised data analysis and critically reviewed the manuscript. All the authors reviewed and approved the final manuscript as submitted and agree to be accountable for all aspects of the work. Y.-C.T. willingly accepted the role of guarantor for this study. All authors have read and agreed to the published version of the manuscript.

Funding: This study was supported by a grant from the Taipei Tzu Chi Hospital, Buddhist Tzu Chi Medical Foundation (Grant No. TCRD-TPE-110-12).

Institutional Review Board Statement: The study was conducted in accordance with the Declaration of Helsinki and approved by the Institutional Review Board of Taipei Tzu Chi Hospital (No. 06-X34-105) on 10 January 2018.

Informed Consent Statement: Patient consent was waived due to the study's retrospective nature, and anonymous clinical data were used for the analysis.

Data Availability Statement: The datasets analyzed during the current study are available from the corresponding author on reasonable request.

Acknowledgments: All members of the Taiwan Upper Tract Urothelial Carcinoma Collaboration group: Allen W. Chiu, Bing-Juin Chiang, Chao-Hsiang Chang, Chao-Yuan Huang, Cheng-Huang Shen, Cheng-Kuang Yang, Cheng-Ling Lee, Chen-Hsun Ho, Che-Wei Chang, Chia-Chang Wu, Chieh-Chun Liao, Chien-Hui Ou, Chih-Chen Hsu, Chih-Chin Yu, Chih-Hung Lin, Chih-Ming Lu, Chih-Yin Yeh, Ching-Chia Li, Chi-Ping Huang, Chi-Rei Yang, Chi-Wen Lo, Chuan-Shu Chen, Chung-Hsin Chen, Chung-You Tsai, Chung-Yu Lin, Chun-Hou Liao, Chun-Kai Hsu, Fang-Yu Ku, Hann-Chorng Kuo, Han-Yu Weng, Hao-Han Chang, Hong-Chiang Chang, Hsiao-Jen Chung, Hsin-Chih Yeh, Hsu-Che Huang, Ian-Seng Cheong, I-Hsuan Alan Chen, Jen-Kai Fang, Jen-Shu Tseng, Jen-Tai Lin, Jian-Hua Hong, Jih-Sheng Chen, Jungle Chi-Hsiang Wu, Kai-Jie Yu, Keng-Kok Tan, Kuan-Hsun Huang, Kun-Lin Hsieh, Lian-Ching Yu, Lun-Hsiang Yuan, Hao-Lun Luo, Marcelo Chen, Min-Hsin Yang, Pai-Yu Cheng, Po-Hung Lin, Richard Chen-Yu Wu, See-Tong Pang, Shin-Hong Chen, Shin-Mei Wong, Shiu-Dong Chung, Shi-Wei Huang, Shuo-Meng Wang, Shu-Yu, Wu, Steven Kuan-Hua Huang, Ta-Yao Tai, Thomas Y. Hsueh, Ting-En Tai, Victor Chia-Hsiang Lin, Wei-Chieh Chen, Wei-Ming Li, Wei-Yu Lin, Wen-Hsin Tseng, Wen-Jeng Wu, Wun-Rong Lin, Yao-Chou Tsai, Yen-Chuan Ou, Yeong-Chin Jou, Yeong-Shiau Pu, Yi-Chia Lin, Yi-Hsuan Wu, Yi-Huei Chang, Yi-sheng Lin, Yi-Sheng Tai, Yu-Khun Lee, Yuan-Hong Jiang, Yu-Che Hsieh, Yu-Chi Chen, Yu-Ching Wen, Yung-Tai Chen, and Zhe-Rui Yang.

Conflicts of Interest: The authors declare no conflicts of interest. The funders had no role in the design of the study; in the collection, analyses, or interpretation of data; in the writing of the manuscript; or in the decision to publish the results.

References

1. Rouprêt, M.; Babjuk, M.; Compérat, E.; Zigeuner, R.; Sylvester, R.J.; Burger, M.; Cowan, N.C.; Gontero, P.; Van Rhijn, B.W.; Mostafid, A.H. European association of urology guidelines on upper urinary tract urothelial carcinoma: 2017 update. *Eur. Urol.* **2018**, *73*, 111–122. [CrossRef] [PubMed]
2. Miyake, M.; Tatsumi, Y.; Fujimoto, K.; Nagao, K.; Sakano, S.; Matsuyama, H.; Inamoto, T.; Azuma, H.; Yasumoto, H.; Shiina, H. Changes in oncological outcomes after radical nephroureterectomy in patients with upper urinary tract urothelial carcinoma

treated in the last two decades: A retrospective analysis based on a multicenter collaborative study. *Jpn. J. Clin. Oncol.* **2016**, *46*, 1148–1155. [CrossRef] [PubMed]

Munoz, J.J.; Ellison, L.M. Upper tract urothelial neoplasms: Incidence and survival during the last 2 decades. *J. Urol.* **2000**, *164*, 1523–1525. [CrossRef] [PubMed]

Yang, M.-H.; Chen, K.-K.; Yen, C.-C.; Wang, W.-S.; Chang, Y.-H.; Huang, W.J.-S.; Fan, F.S.; Chiou, T.-J.; Liu, J.-H.; Chen, P.-M. Unusually high incidence of upper urinary tract urothelial carcinoma in Taiwan. *Urology* **2002**, *59*, 681–687. [CrossRef]

Chou, Y.H.; Huang, C.H. Unusual clinical presentation of upper urothelial carcinoma in Taiwan. *Cancer* **1999**, *85*, 1342–1344. [CrossRef]

Siegel, R.L.; Miller, K.D.; Jemal, A. Cancer statistics, 2018. *CA A Cancer J. Clin.* **2018**, *68*, 7–30. [CrossRef]

Chiang, C.-J.; Lo, W.-C.; Yang, Y.-W.; You, S.-L.; Chen, C.-J.; Lai, M.-S. Incidence and survival of adult cancer patients in Taiwan, 2002–2012. *J. Formos. Med. Assoc.* **2016**, *115*, 1076–1088. [CrossRef]

Margulis, V.; Shariat, S.F.; Matin, S.F.; Kamat, A.M.; Zigeuner, R.; Kikuchi, E.; Lotan, Y.; Weizer, A.; Raman, J.D.; Wood, C.G. Outcomes of radical nephroureterectomy: A series from the Upper Tract Urothelial Carcinoma Collaboration. *Cancer* **2009**, *115*, 1224–1233. [CrossRef]

Reddy, K.; Gharde, P.; Tayade, H.; Patil, M.; Reddy, L.S.; Surya, D. Advancements in robotic surgery: A comprehensive overview of current utilizations and upcoming frontiers. *Cureus* **2023**, *15*, e50415. [CrossRef]

10. Tinay, I.; Gelpi-Hammerschmidt, F.; Leow, J.J.; Allard, C.B.; Rodriguez, D.; Wang, Y.; Chung, B.I.; Chang, S.L. Trends in utilisation, perioperative outcomes, and costs of nephroureterectomies in the management of upper tract urothelial carcinoma: A 10-year population-based analysis. *BJU Int.* **2016**, *117*, 954–960. [CrossRef]
11. Grossmann, N.C.; Soria, F.; Juvet, T.; Potretzke, A.M.; Djaladat, H.; Ghoreifi, A.; Kikuchi, E.; Mari, A.; Khene, Z.-E.; Fujita, K. Comparing oncological and perioperative outcomes of open versus laparoscopic versus robotic radical nephroureterectomy for the treatment of upper tract urothelial carcinoma: A multicenter, multinational, propensity score-matched analysis. *Cancers* **2023**, *15*, 1409. [CrossRef] [PubMed]
12. Mourmouris, P.; ARGUN, Ö.; Tzelves, L.; Tuna, M.; Gourtzelidou, M.; Tziotis, A.; Kural, A.; Skolarikos, A. Is robotic radical nephroureterectomy a safe alternative to open approach: The first prospective analysis. *Arch. Ital. Urol. Androl.* **2021**, *93*, 4. [CrossRef] [PubMed]
13. Zeuschner, P.; Vollmer, S.G.; Linxweiler, J.; Wagenpfeil, G.; Wagenpfeil, S.; Saar, M.; Siemer, S.; Stöckle, M.; Heinzelbecker, J. Robot-assisted versus open radical nephroureterectomy for urothelial carcinoma of the upper urinary tract: A retrospective cohort study across ten years. *Surg. Oncol.* **2021**, *38*, 101607. [CrossRef]
14. Ambani, S.N.; Weizer, A.Z.; Wolf, J.S., Jr.; He, C.; Miller, D.C.; Montgomery, J.S. Matched comparison of robotic vs laparoscopic nephroureterectomy: An initial experience. *Urology* **2014**, *83*, 345–349. [CrossRef] [PubMed]
15. Hu, C.-Y.; Yang, C.-K.; Huang, C.-Y.; Ou, Y.-C.; Hung, S.-F.; Chung, S.-D.; Pu, Y.-S. Robot-assisted laparoscopic nephroureterectomy versus hand-assisted laparoscopic nephroureterectomy for upper urinary tract urothelial carcinoma: A matched comparison study. *BioMed Res. Int.* **2015**, *2015*, 918486. [CrossRef]
16. Melquist, J.J.; Redrow, G.; Delacroix, S.; Park, A.; Faria, E.E.; Karam, J.A.; Matin, S.F. Comparison of single-docking robotic-assisted and traditional laparoscopy for retroperitoneal lymph node dissection during nephroureterectomy with bladder cuff excision for upper-tract urothelial carcinoma. *Urology* **2016**, *87*, 216–223. [CrossRef]
17. Li, C.-C.; Chang, C.-H.; Huang, C.-P.; Hong, J.-H.; Huang, C.-Y.; Chen, I.-H.A.; Lin, J.-T.; Lo, C.-W.; Yu, C.-C.; Tseng, J.-S. Comparing oncological outcomes and surgical complications of hand-assisted, laparoscopic and robotic nephroureterectomy for upper tract urothelial carcinoma. *Front. Oncol.* **2021**, *11*, 731460. [CrossRef]
18. Pearce, S.M.; Pariser, J.J.; Patel, S.G.; Steinberg, G.D.; Shalhav, A.L.; Smith, N.D. The effect of surgical approach on performance of lymphadenectomy and perioperative morbidity for radical nephroureterectomy. *Urol. Oncol. Semin. Orig. Investig.* **2016**, *34*, 121.e115–121.e121. [CrossRef]
19. Lenis, A.T.; Donin, N.M.; Faiena, I.; Salmasi, A.; Johnson, D.C.; Drakaki, A.; Gollapudi, K.; Blumberg, J.; Belldegrun, A.; Pantuck, A. Role of surgical approach on lymph node dissection yield and survival in patients with upper tract urothelial carcinoma. *Urol. Oncol. Semin. Orig. Investig.* **2018**, *36*, 9.e1–9.e9. [CrossRef]
20. Friedman, J. The Elements of Statistical Learning: Data Mining, Inference, and Prediction. 2009. Available online: https://hastie.su.domains/ElemStatLearn/ (accessed on 19 April 2025).
21. Thomas, L.E.; Li, F.; Pencina, M.J. Overlap weighting: A propensity score method that mimics attributes of a randomized clinical trial. *JAMA* **2020**, *323*, 2417–2418. [CrossRef]
22. Cheng, C.; Li, F.; Thomas, L.E.; Li, F. Addressing extreme propensity scores in estimating counterfactual survival functions via the overlap weights. *Am. J. Epidemiol.* **2022**, *191*, 1140–1151. [CrossRef] [PubMed]

23. Ashrafian, H.; Clancy, O.; Grover, V.; Darzi, A. The evolution of robotic surgery: Surgical and anaesthetic aspects. *BJA Br. Anaesth.* **2017**, *119*, i72–i84. [CrossRef] [PubMed]
24. Castilho, T.M.L.; Lemos, G.C.; Cha, J.D.; Colombo, J.R.; Claros, O.R.; Lemos, M.B.; Carneiro, A. Transition from open parti nephrectomy directly to robotic surgery: Experience of a single surgeon to achieve "TRIFECTA". *Int. Braz. J. Urol.* **2020**, *4* 814–821. [CrossRef] [PubMed]
25. Ghani, K.R.; Sukumar, S.; Sammon, J.D.; Rogers, C.G.; Trinh, Q.-D.; Menon, M. Practice patterns and outcomes of open an minimally invasive partial nephrectomy since the introduction of robotic partial nephrectomy: Results from the nationwid inpatient sample. *J. Urol.* **2014**, *191*, 907–913. [CrossRef]
26. Patel, M.N.; Bhandari, M.; Menon, M.; Rogers, C.G. Robotic-assisted partial nephrectomy. *BJU Int.* **2009**, *103*, 1296–131 [CrossRef]
27. Chatterjee, S.; Das, S.; Ganguly, K.; Mandal, D. Advancements in robotic surgery: Innovations, challenges and future prospects. *Robot. Surg.* **2024**, *18*, 28. [CrossRef]
28. Tyson II, M.D.; Andrews, P.E.; Ferrigni, R.F.; Humphreys, M.R.; Parker, A.S.; Castle, E.P. Radical prostatectomy trends in th United States: 1998 to 2011. *Mayo Clin. Proc.* **2016**, *91*, 10–16. [CrossRef]
29. Morriss, S.; Zargar, H.; Dias, B.H. Management of the distal ureter during nephroureterectomy for upper tract urothelia carcinoma: A comprehensive review of literature. *Urol. J.* **2021**, *18*, 585–599.
30. Xylinas, E.; Colin, P.; Audenet, F.; Phe, V.; Cormier, L.; Cussenot, O.; Houlgatte, A.; Karsenty, G.; Bruyère, F.; Polguer, Intravesical recurrence after radical nephroureterectomy for upper tract urothelial carcinomas: Predictors and impact o subsequent oncological outcomes from a national multicenter study. *World J. Urol.* **2013**, *31*, 61–68. [CrossRef]
31. Braun, A.E.; Srivastava, A.; Maffucci, F.; Kutikov, A. Controversies in management of the bladder cuff at nephroureterectom *Transl. Androl. Urol.* **2020**, *9*, 1868. [CrossRef]
32. Lee, H.; Kim, H.J.; Lee, S.E.; Hong, S.K.; Byun, S.-S. Comparison of oncological and perioperative outcomes of open, laparoscopi and robotic nephroureterectomy approaches in patients with non-metastatic upper-tract urothelial carcinoma. *PLoS ONE* **201** *14*, e0210401. [CrossRef] [PubMed]
33. Yu, C.-C.; Chen, C.-H.; Hong, J.-H.; Ke, H.-L.; Li, W.-M.; Chung, S.-D.; Wu, W.-C.; Chen, Y.-T.; Jiang, Y.-H.; Lin, Y.-H. Compariso of oncological outcomes for hand-assisted and pure laparoscopic radical nephroureterectomy: Results from the Taiwan Uppe Tract Urothelial Cancer Collaboration Group. *Surg. Endosc.* **2022**, *36*, 4342–4434. [CrossRef] [PubMed]
34. Kitamura, H.; Maeda, T.; Tanaka, T.; Fukuta, F.; Kobayashi, K.; Nishiyama, N.; Takahashi, S.; Masumori, N. Comparison o laparoscopic, hand-assisted, and open surgical nephroureterectomy. *JSLS J. Soc. Laparoendosc. Surg.* **2014**, *18*, 288. [CrossRef]
35. Ji, R.; He, Z.; Fang, S.; Yang, W.; Wei, M.; Dong, J.; Xu, W.; Ji, Z. Robot-assisted vs. laparoscopic nephroureterectomy for uppe urinary tract urothelial carcinoma: A systematic review and meta-analysis based on comparative studies. *Front. Oncol.* **2022** *12*, 964256. [CrossRef] [PubMed]
36. Jeong, I.G.; Khandwala, Y.S.; Kim, J.H.; Han, D.H.; Li, S.; Wang, Y.; Chang, S.L.; Chung, B.I. Association of robotic-assisted vs laparoscopic radical nephrectomy with perioperative outcomes and health care costs, 2003 to 2015. *JAMA* **2017**, *318*, 1561–1568. [CrossRef]
37. Peng, L.; Mehmud, I.; Meng, C.; Tang, D.; Li, K.; Gan, L.; Li, J.; Yi, F.; Li, Y. Comparison of perioperative outcomes and complications of laparoscopic and robotic nephroureterectomy approaches in patients with upper-tract urothelial carcinoma. *Ann. Surg. Oncol.* **2023**, *30*, 3805–3816. [CrossRef]

cancers

MDPI

Systematic Review

Adrenalectomy Performed with the Da Vinci Single-Port Robotic System: A Systematic Review and Pooled Analysis

Giuseppe Reitano [1], Arianna Tumminello [1], Carlo Prevato [1], Anna Cacco [1], Greta Gaggiato [1], Giorgia Baù [1], Lorenzo Sabato [1], Elisa Tonet [1], Anna Gambarotto [1], Valerio Fusca [1], Kevin Martina [1], Silvia Visentin [1], Giovanni Betto [1], Giacomo Novara [1], Fabrizio Dal Moro [1] and Fabio Zattoni [1,2,*]

1 Department of Surgery, Oncology and Gastroenterology (DISCOG), University of Padova, 35128 Padova, Italy
2 Department of Medicine (DIMED), University of Padova, 35128 Padova, Italy
* Correspondence: fabio.zattoni@unipd.it

Simple Summary: Da Vinci Single-Port surgery is rapidly gaining adoption worldwide. Adrenalectomy provides an ideal context for the implementation of the Da Vinci Single-Port system. Single-port adrenalectomy appears to be both feasible and safe, potentially offering excellent cosmetic outcomes and reduced hospital stays.

Abstract: Introduction: The Da Vinci Single-Port (DV-SP) system emerged in 2018 but there is limited evidence on its use and perioperative outcomes for robot-assisted adrenalectomy (RAA). Methods: A systematic search was performed through PubMed, Scopus, Ovid, and WoS in December 2024. A PICO framework was used. Population: adult patients with adrenal masses; Intervention: DV-SP RAA; Outcomes: feasibility, reproducibility and safety of DV-SP RAA. A total of five retrospective studies involving 342 patients were included. The quantitative analysis was conducted using a random-effect model or a fixed-effect model as appropriate. A risk of bias assessment for non-randomized comparative studies and case series was performed. Results: The pooled mean operative time was 92.5 min (95% confidence interval [CI] 71.2, 113.9, p $I^2 = 0\%$, four studies), and the mean estimated blood loss (EBL) was 26.5 mL (95%CI −8.1, 61.2, $I^2 = 98.2\%$, three studies). Most of the procedures were completed with a single incision, though some required additional port placement, with a proportion of 9% (95%CI 0, 29, $I^2 = 71.7\%$, five studies). Perioperative complications were rare (0%, 95% CI 0, 4, $I^2 = 0\%$, five studies). Two studies comparing DV-SP and DV multi-port (MP) found no significant differences in complications. One study compared DV-SP RAA to DV Si or Xi single-access procedures. DV-SP showed improved operative techniques and better cosmetic outcomes. Limitations of this study are small sample size and potential selection bias due to smaller masses in the DV-SP RAA group. Conclusions: DV-SP RAA is a promising approach, offering reduced operative time, low EBL, and excellent cosmetic results. This study shows that DV-SP RAA seems reproducible, feasible, and safe. Limitation of the included studies are small sample size and selection bias, which limits the generalizability of the results. Randomized comparative studies between DV-SP and MP RAA are needed to further validate these findings.

Keywords: Da Vinci Single-Port; robot-assisted adrenalectomy; laparoscopic adrenalectomy; single-site surgery; adrenal masses

1. Introduction

Adrenal masses encompass a variety of tumors, most of which are benign, though some can be malignant. A portion of benign adrenal masses may secrete excess hormones, but the majority (71–84%) are non-functional adenomas, often found incidentally on imaging [1]. Hormone-secreting adenomas can produce a variety of cortical and medullary hormones, including cortisol, aldosterone, and catecholamines. Malignant tumors may be metastases from other solid tumors (such as lung or kidney cancer) or primary adrenal cortical cancers. Primary adrenal cancers are rare but aggressive and present distinctive features, such as high Hounsfield units (6.3% of adrenal masses are malignant when HU >20) [2] or rapid growth (>3 mm/year) [3].

Adrenalectomy, when indicated, can be performed using either a minimally invasive technique (laparoscopy or robotic surgery) or through traditional open surgery. The latter is typically preferred for larger tumors (>6–8 cm) suspected of being adrenocortical carcinoma, as well as for those with CT evidence of local invasion [4].

Over the past 30 years, laparoscopic adrenalectomy (LA) has been the approach of choice for the surgical removal of adrenal adenomas, offering shorter hospital stay and fewer complications compared to the open approach [5]. Since its approval, the Da Vinci-Multi-Port (DV-MP) system (Intuitive, Sunnyvale, CA, USA) has been utilized for adrenalectomy, due to its ability to perform complex minimally invasive operations and to reduce the morbidity, the size and the number of incisions [6]. Robotic-assisted adrenalectomy (RAA) yields similar outcomes in terms of operative time, complications, and oncological results when compared to LA [7]. However, RAA offers enhanced ergonomics; a 3D view; tremor filtration; and superior range of motion, flexibility, and precision [8]. At the same time, RAA appears to be safer for obese patients (BMI > 30 kg/m^2), with a lower conversion rate compared to LA [9]. Further, the robotic approach may offer a safer option for larger masses (>6 cm), as the mean operative time seems shorter with RAA compared to laparoscopic surgery [10]. However, high costs and the limited availability of robotic platforms may be significant disadvantages of RAA [9]. The development and spread of more affordable robotic platforms could present an opportunity to reduce costs and enhance the performance of RAA [11].

The evolution of robotic surgery to a single point of access may further reduce pain and potentially reduce the hospital stay [12]. The Da Vinci Single-Port (DV-SP) system uses a single arm to deliver three multi-jointed instruments and a fully wristed 3D high-definition camera through a single 2.5 cm cannula. Since gaining FDA approval in 2018, several high-volume centers have reported their experience using DV-SP for a variety of urologic procedures, including radical prostatectomy [13], simple prostatectomy [14], partial nephrectomy [15], colposacropexy [16], and pyeloplasty [17]. However, evidence regarding DV-SP use and perioperative outcomes for adrenalectomy remains limited. Significant challenges in terms of maneuverability, tissue retraction, and working space remain with the DV-SP, creating a unique learning curve compared to the DV-MP. This systematic review aims to provide a comprehensive understanding of the feasibility, reproducibility, and safety of DV-SP RAA.

2. Materials and Methods

2.1. Search Strategy

The study protocol was registered in the International Prospective Register of Ongoing Systematic Review in Health and Social Care (PROSPERO ID: CRD42023451162). In adherence with the Preferred Reporting Items for Systematic Review and Meta-Analyses (PRISMA) [18], a systematic search was conducted in December 2024 through PubMed, Scopus, Ovid, and Web of Science. The search strategy included the following terms "robot*" AND "single port" AND "adrenalectomy". Only papers written in English were retained.

2.2. Inclusion Criteria, Exclusion Criteria, and Outcomes

A PICO framework was used to formulate research questions and inclusion and exclusion criteria [19]. The population of interest was composed of adult patients with adrenal masses undergoing DV-SP RAA (intervention). Laparoscopy, multiport robotic systems, and non-DV single-port devices were allowed as comparative arms (comparator). The primary outcomes of the study were feasibility, reproducibility, and safety of DV-SP RAA. Clinical trials, prospective and retrospective cohort studies, and case–control studies focusing on DV SP RAA and exploring at least one of the outcomes of interest were included. Animal models, studies on children, dry and wet lab experiences, conference abstracts, posters, editorials, and letters were excluded. Only the most recent publications were retained, and older manuscripts were excluded if data overlapped. References from the manuscript included for the full text analysis were also screened.

2.3. Selection Process and Data Extraction

Two authors (G.R. and A.T.) independently screened and identified relevant articles for the full text analysis using Covidence (Veritas Health Innovation, Melbourne, Australia). Data from the articles selected after the full text review were collected using Microsoft Excel (Redmond, Washington, DC, USA). The information collected was demographics, operative time, estimated blood loss (EBL), need for blood transfusions, length of stay (LoS) early and late post-operative complications according to Clavien–Dindo classification [20], postoperative pain, and positive surgical margins (PSM). Screening and data abstraction were verified by a third author (F.Z.) who was also involved in conflict resolution.

2.4. Risk of Bias Assessment

Risk of bias (RoB) was assessed through the ROBINS-I for non-randomized studies [21], and European Association of Urology (EAU) guidelines for systematic case series review [22] were used for the only non-comparative study. RoB assessment was carried out by two independent reviewers (A.T. and A.C.) and verified by a third author (F.Z.).

2.5. Statistical Analysis

A narrative synthesis of the studies was provided alongside a quantitative analysis. Pooled effects and 95% confidence intervals (95%CI) were obtained using the mean and standard deviation for continuous variables [23], while binary and categorical variables were summarized using the inverse-variance method. Event rates with 95%CI were calculated using the Freeman–Tukey double-arcsine transformation to stabilize the variance of the reported proportions. Chi-square-based Q test and I^2 statistics were used to assess whether there was significant heterogeneity across studies. Based on heterogeneity, a meta-analysis was performed using either a random-effects model (REM, $I^2 > 50\%$) or a fixed-effects model (FEM, $I^2 \leq 50\%$). The DerSimonian–Laird estimator was used to estimate between-study variance for binary and categorical variables. Forrest plots were used to graphically display the main results. A significance threshold of p-value < 0.05 was applied to determine statistical significance for the overall effect size. All analyses were conducted using STATA version 18.0 (StataCorp, College Station, TX, USA, 2023).

3. Results

3.1. Study Selection, Characteristics, and Quality

After a systematic literature search, 274 articles were identified. Duplicates were removed either automatically using Covidence or manually. Articles that did not meet the inclusion criteria were excluded after the initial screening. Following a full-text review, five articles [12,24–27] involving 342 patients in total and 72 patients undergoing DV-SP RAA were included in the evidence synthesis (Figure 1). Only one study was excluded from the quantitative analysis of continuous variables due to aggregated data but was retained for the analysis of categorical and binary variables. According to the RoB assessment, all the comparative studies were considered to have a high-risk of bias (Figure 2). The only case-series was also at high risk of bias due to selection of participants without clear inclusion and exclusion criteria.

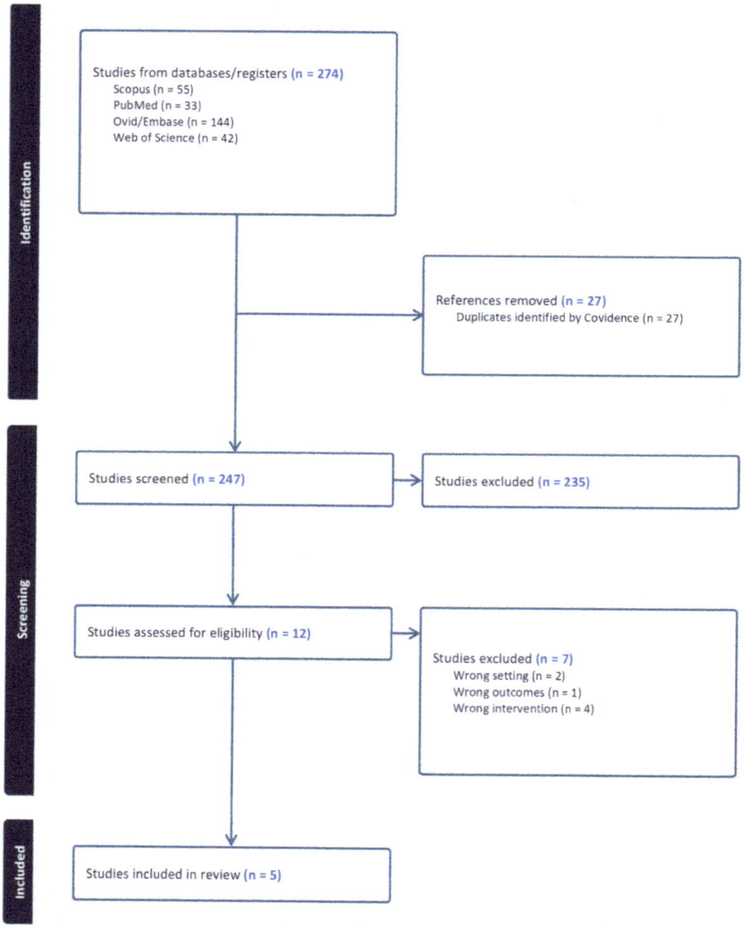

Figure 1. PRISMA flow-chart.

3.2. Patient Characteristics

Baseline, intra-operative, and postoperative features are summarized in Table 1. The pooled median age was 49 years (95%CI 38.7, 59.2, $I^2 = 0\%$), and body mass index (BMI) was 26.8 kg/m^2 (95%CI 22.9, 30.8, $I^2 = 0\%$). The most common systemic syndrome associated with the presence of the adrenal mass was primary hyperaldosteronism (26/68, 38%) followed by pheochromocytoma syndrome (11/68, 16%). Incidentalomas were frequent, with 19 (28%) cases among the 4 studies included in the pooled analysis.

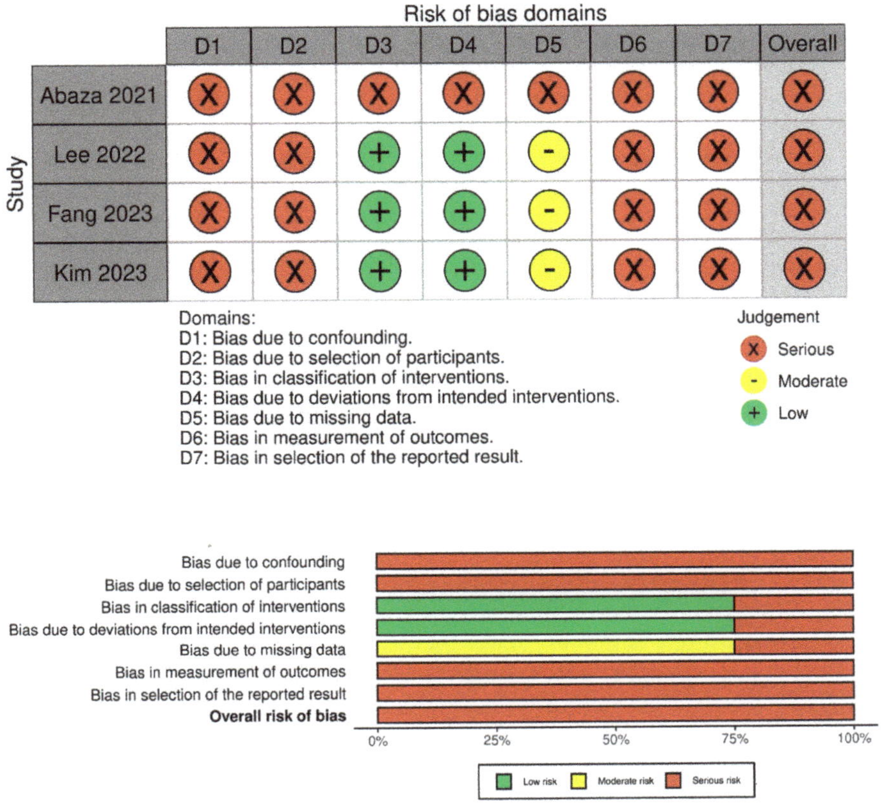

Figure 2. Comparative studies [12,24–26]—Risk of Bias Assessment (ROBINS-I).

Table 1. Baseline characteristics. BMI: body mass index; SD: standard deviation.

Author, Year	Study Design	Country	Robot	Number of Patients	Sex n (%)	BMI (Kg/m^2) Mean (SD)	Prior Abdominal Surgeries n (%)	Adrenal Mass Diameter (cm) Mean (SD)
Rudnick 2024 [27]	Case series	USA	Da Vinci Single-Port	19	M: 10 (52.6) F: 9 (47.4)	31 (4.5)	13 (68.4)	5.2 (3.9)
Fang 2023 [25]	Case–control	USA	Da Vinci Single-Port	11	M: 3 (27.3) F: 8 (72.7)	31.8 (5.9)	8 (72.7)	2.8 (1.3)
			Da Vinci Multi-Port	25	M: 12 (48%) F: 13 (52%)	32 (8.3)	15 (60)	4.1 (1.8)
Kim 2023 [26]	Case–control	Korea	Da Vinci Single-Port	30	M: 12 (40) F: 18 (60)	24.7 (3.9)	-	2.1 (1)
			Da Vinci Multi-Port (3 ports)	117	M: 41 (35.2) F: 76 (64.8)	24.6 (3.6)	-	3.9 (2.7)
			Da Vinci Multi-Port (2 ports)	103	M: 32 (31) F: 71 (69)	25.2 (5.4)	-	3 (1.4)
Lee 2022 [24]	Case–control	Korea	Da Vinci Single-Port	8	M: 4 (50) F: 4 (50)	24.8 (3.1)	2/8 (25)	1.7 (1)
			Da Vinci Multi-Port	11	M: 4 (36.4) F: 7 (63.6)	22.2 (1.8)	3/11 (27.2)	2.3 (1.9)
Abaza 2021 [12]	Case–control	Ireland	Da Vinci Single-Port	4	-	-	-	-
			Da Vinci Multi-Port	14	-	-	-	-

The pooled adrenal mass diameter was 2.2 cm (95%CI 1, 3.4, $I^2 = 0\%$).

3.3. Surgical Outcomes Associated with DV-SP RAA

Surgical outcomes can be reviewed in Table 2. Retroperitoneal DV-SP RAA was performed in 37 cases (51.4%) [24,26], while 35 (48.6%) adrenalectomies were completed using a transperitoneal approach [12,24,25,27]. Three studies [24,25,27] reported prior abdominal surgeries, accounting for a total of 23 cases.

Table 2. Perioperative outcomes. SD: standard deviation; EBL: estimated blood loss; C-D: Clavien–Dindo; PSM: positive surgical margins.

Author, Year	Robot	Total Operative Time (min) Mean (SD)	Docking Time (min) Mean (SD)	Console Time (min) Mean (SD)	Additional Assistant Port Required n (%)	EBL (mL) Mean (SD)	Perioperative Complications n (%)	Conversion to Open n (%)	PSM n (%)
Rudnick 2024 [27]	Da Vinci Single-Port	80.7 (22.9)	7.6 (2)	68 (12.6)	2/19 (10.5)	63.9 (52)	C-D < 3: 2/19 (10.5) C-D ≥ 3: 1/19 (5)	0/19 (0)	1/19 (5)
Fang 2023 [25]	Da Vinci Single-Port	124.6 (38.5)	-	-	5/11 (45.4)	18.1 (13)	C-D ≥ 3: 0/11 (0)	0/11 (0)	1/11 (9)
	Da Vinci Multi-Port	146.4 (48.1)	-	-	-	65.6 (95)	C-D ≥ 3: 1/25 (4)	0/25 (0)	0/25 (0)
Kim 2023 [26]	Da Vinci Single-Port	80.9 (22.1)	-	-	0/30 (0)	-	C-D ≥ 1: 0/30 (0)	0/30 (0)	-
	Da Vinci Multi-Port (3 ports)	134.6 (65.8)	-	-	-	-	C-D ≥ 1: 4/117 (3.4)	0/117 (0)	-
	Da Vinci Multi-Port (2 ports)	99.9 (27.6)	-	-	-	-	C-D ≥ 1: 1/103 (1)	0/103 (0)	-
Lee 2022 [24]	Da Vinci Single-Port	99 (16.2)	4.8 (2.4)	57.1 (15.2)	1/8 (12.5)	2.5 (4.6)	C-D ≥ 1: 0/8 (0)	0/8 (0)	-
	Da Vinci Multi-Port	121.9 (50.7)	7.7 (4.4)	49.1 (10.6)	-	17.3 (18.5)	C-D ≥ 1: 0/11 (0)	0/11 (0) *	-
Abaza 2020 [12]	Da Vinci Single-Port	106.4 **	-	-	0/4 (0)	-	0/4 (0)	0/4 (0)	-

* Two surgeries were completed through a laparoscopic approach. ** Data aggregated with partial cystectomy, nephrectomy, and nephroureterectomy.

Patients were placed either in a lateral decubitus [25], a prone jackknife position with flexion of the hip joint for retroperitoneal access [24,26], or a modified flank position with a slight flexion [27]. For the retroperitoneal approach, all authors employed a 3 cm transverse incision just beneath the tip of the 12th rib [24,26]. For the transperitoneal approach, Rudnick et al. initially used a 3 cm supraumbilical incision [27], which was later modified to a lower quadrant incision, positioned two-thirds of the way between the umbilicus and the iliac crest, while Fang et al. used a 2 cm incision on the lateral side of the umbilicus [25].

Pooled total operative time was 92.5 min (95%CI 71.2, 113.9, $I^2 = 0\%$, Figure 3A).

Most of the procedures were completed with a single incision, though some required the placement of an additional port. In three studies, an additional 5–8 mm assistant port was placed in 2 (10%) [27], 1 (12.5%) [24], and 5 (45.4%) [25] of SP cases for suction, irrigation, and retraction, and to aid in dissection. Abaza et al. [12] and Kim et al. [26] successfully performed 100% of the procedures with single access. The pooled proportion of the additional port required was 9% (95%CI 0, 29, $I^2 = 71.7\%$, Figure 3C).

The mean EBL was 26.5 mL (95%CI −8.1, 61.2, $I^2 = 98.2\%$, Figure 3B).

Conversion to open surgery or laparoscopy was not required in any case [12,24–27].

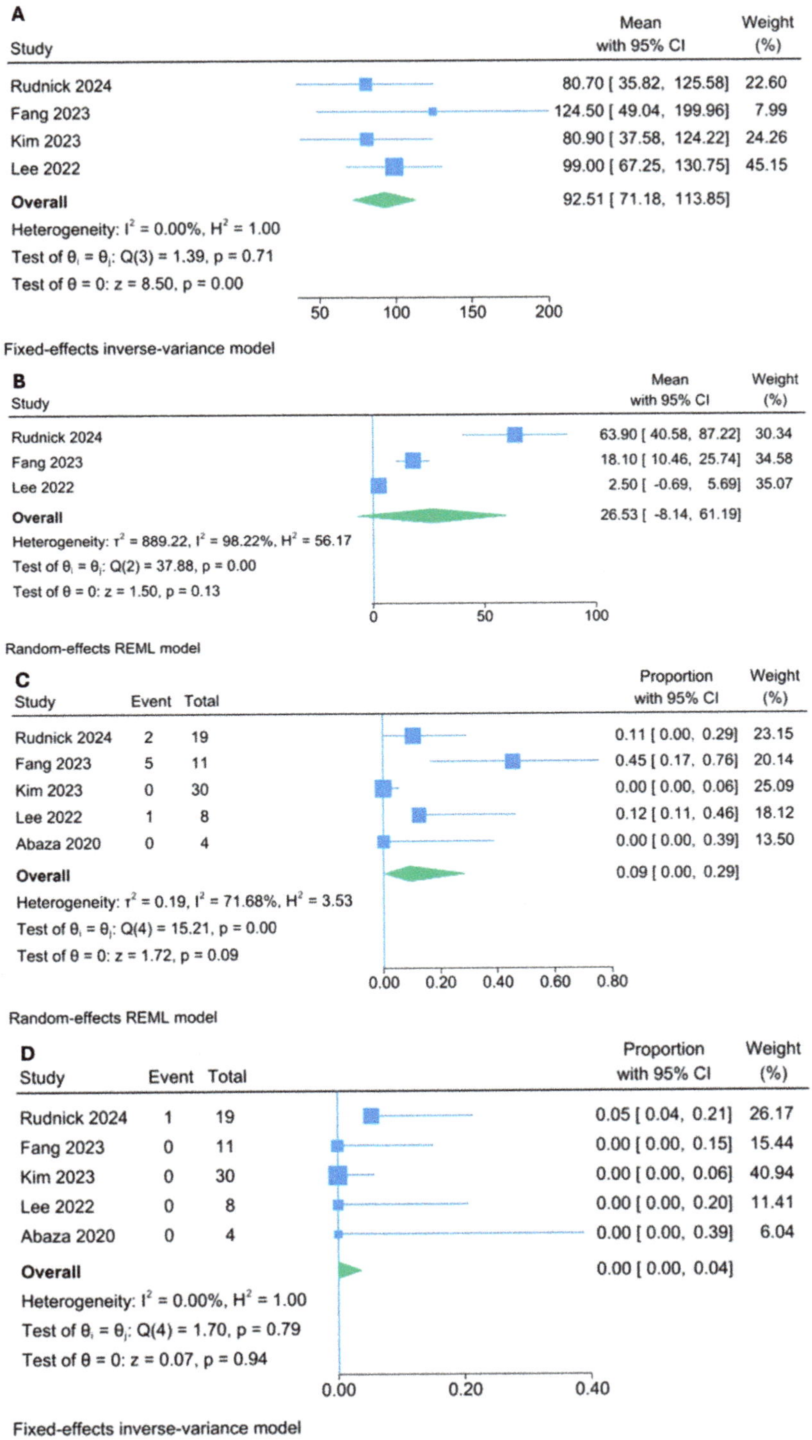

Figure 3. (**A**) total operative time; (**B**) estimated blood loss; (**C**) additional port placement; (**D**) complications Clavien–Dindo ≥ IIIa [12,24–27].

High-grade perioperative complications (Clavien–Dindo ≥ III) were rare (0%, 95% CI 0, 4, I^2 = 0%, Figure 3D). In the study by Rudnick et al. [27], two grade II Clavien–Dindo complications (paralytic ileus and hypotension due to adrenal insufficiency managed with steroids) and one grade IIIb Clavien–Dindo complication was reported. The only high-grade complication, identified on postoperative day 6, involved a sepsis with transient ipsilateral ureteropelvic junction (UPJ) obstruction due to edema near the UPJ, which required the placement of a ureteral stent for 6 weeks. No other high-grade complications were described in the DV-SP arm [12,24–26].

Postoperative pain evaluated using a numeric rating scale the day of surgery was available only in two studies with means (averaged over the first six hours postoperatively) of 3.7 (0–8) [12] and 5.3 (±1.1) [26].

Same-day discharge (SDD) was achieved in 100% of the DV-SP surgeries performed by Abaza et al. [12] and Fang et al. [25]. In the other cases, LoS did not exceed 5 days [24,26,27].

PSM were reported in one patient from the series by Rudnick et al. (5.3%) [27] and one from the cases by Fang et al. (9%) [25]. Complete resection was achieved in all cases in the RAA by Kim et al. [26].

3.4. Comparison Between DV-SP and Two-Port or Three-Port DV-MP

Controversial results were observed in terms of operative time. DV-SP RAA seemed to offer shorter operative time in the study by Kim et al. when compared to conventional DV-MP, and this difference was also confirmed when DV-SP RAA was compared to a reduced two-port DV-MP approach (using a multiaccess glove port and a second robotic arm port) [26]. However, in the study by Fang et al., no significant differences were found in terms of operative time between the two approaches [25].

On the other hand, EBL was slightly higher in the MP group [12,25].

No significant differences in major complications were found in the comparative studies between DV-SP and DV-MP RAA [12,25]. Moreover, the only high-grade complication reported by Fang et al. was due to a pneumoperitoneum in the DV-MP arm, which required a surgical drain placement (Clavien–Dindo IIIb) [25].

In DV-SP patients, Abaza et al. [12] reported lower mean pain scores (3.7 vs. 4.5, $p = 0.017$), whereas Kim et al. did not find a significant difference in immediate postoperative pain scores (5.3 vs. 5.3 vs. 5.8, $p = 0.958$) [26].

SDD was less common among DV-MP RAA procedures in the surgeries performed by Abaza et al., with only 79% of patients discharged the same day [12]. However, among cases treated at the University of Ulsan College of Medicine, 100% of patients undergoing RAA were discharged the same day, regardless of the approach used (SP or MP) [26].

3.5. Comparison Between DV-SP and Single-Port Access DV-MP

Lee et al. compared DV-SP with DV-MP (Si or Xi) using a single-port access (SA) [24].

No significant differences were observed in operative and console time. Although statistical significance was not reached for docking time, a difference of 2.6 min was noted. Estimated blood loss (EBL) was similar between groups, and no perioperative complications were observed. The length of stay was 2.5 ± 0.5 days for DV-SP patients and 3.4 ± 1.1 days for SA RAA patients. Conversion to laparoscopy was required in only two (18.2%) cases among patients undergoing SA RAA, while an additional port for liver retraction was needed in the only transperitoneal DV-SP RAA case (a patient with a 3.7 cm tumor). The scar aspect was better with DV-SP RAA, as the incision size in SA-RAA patients was increased by the tension from surgical arm movements.

4. Discussion

The field of RAA is rapidly expanding with the introduction of several new platforms that may, in the future, offer comparable operative outcomes to the standard DV-MP [11]. In this context, DV-SP RAA, introduced in 2018, has shown feasibility, safety, and effectiveness based on early published experiences. This approach seems to yield satisfactory surgical and pathological outcomes, making it a promising advancement in the field.

Compared to SA laparoscopic and robotic surgery, DV-SP offers distinct advantages, including a flexible camera with a three-dimensional magnified view and a three-articulated, multi-jointed working arm. These features coming through a 2.5 cm cannula enhance movement efficiency and allow for more precise and fluid surgical operations. In contrast, DV-MP RAA with SA is constrained by arm collisions and often necessitates an additional port for the assistant [24]. DV-SP mitigates these issues by minimizing arm interference and reducing the assistant's role at the operative table. A key distinction from DV-MP is that, while DV-MP relies on individual wrist rotations for each arm, DV-SP enables movement up to the wrist and elbow within the operative field.

According to a prior systematic review [28], the mean total operative time for laparoscopic RAA was 149.6 min, with a mean pooled estimated blood loss (EBL) of 85.3 mL. For DV-MP RAA, the mean total operative time was 157.2 min, and the mean pooled EBL was 66.9 mL. While a direct quantitative comparison remains challenging, our findings suggest promising performance for RAA with DV-SP.

The remarkably low mean EBL observed may be attributed to the absence of efficient intraoperative bleeding control by energy devices, necessitating meticulous dissection to prevent bleeding and precise vessel clipping. The observed reduction in total operative time may be attributed to the ease of robotic access and the reduced-port design, which generally shortens the time needed for port placement and docking, as well as smoother surgical movements with fewer collisions. However, given that early experiences with DV-SP should logically lead to longer operative time due to the learning curve associated with a new robotic platform, selection bias may have played a role in the observed efficiency. Additionally, extensive prior experience with SA laparoscopy and DV-MP may have facilitated a faster adaptation process for surgeons, allowing them to achieve proficiency with DV-SP more quickly. This was seen in the study by Kim et al. where the learning curve of DV-SP was compared to a standard three-port and a reduced two-port approach [26]. Operative time was shorter for DV-SP even in the earliest cases without a running curve during the learning process.

Also, previous experience with DV-SP may be helpful. For instance, Rudnick et al. reported the lowest mean operative time, likely due to their extensive SP robotic experience, having performed over 600 single-port robotic procedures since 2019 [27].

Regarding complications, our pooled estimate suggests a very low rate. A recent systematic review reported complication rates of 4.8% for robotic RAA and 3.9% for laparoscopic RAA [28]. In terms of LoS, DV-SP has demonstrated potential for increasing the number of same-day discharges (SDD) in selected cases, thereby reducing healthcare costs and the risk of nosocomial infections [12]. Indeed, despite offering greater safety, inpatient management is not necessary for all patients undergoing RAA [29]. Patient selection for SDD should involve a careful evaluation of the patient's psychological and social background, especially in those requiring replacement therapy [29]. This is essential to prevent non-compliance with hormonal treatment, which can result in death or severe postoperative complications due to adrenal insufficiency [29]. Additionally, SDD should be based on a structured program of postoperative evaluations. For example, the Cosyntropin stimulation test should be performed on postoperative day 1 to assess the need for glucocorticoid replacement in patients treated for glucocorticoid-secreting tumors [30]. The program should also include office visits, telemedicine consultations, and the use of wireless sensors to monitor the patient's vital signs outside the hospital [31].

Pooled PSM rates with DV-SP appear to be lower compared to those reported for DV-MP RAA, where the PSM rate was 11% [28]. However, the evaluation of PSM was constrained by limited available data and the predominance of highly selected small tumors, which inherently lower the risk for PSM.

From a cosmetic perspective, DV-SP may offer superior aesthetic outcomes compared to SA surgery [24,26]. As demonstrated by Lee et al., the scar appearance was more favorable with DV-SP RAA, whereas the arm movements required in MP-DV could lead to enlargement of the surgical incision [24].

Postoperative pain and analgesic use after DV-SP RAA were not consistently reported across the studies involved [12,24,26]. It is unclear whether single-port RAA can reduce postoperative pain, and this becomes even more complex when considering the use of different methods to assess postoperative pain and various painkillers, which could compromise the assessment of this outcome.

No data are currently available on disease recurrence after DV-SP RAA, so conclusions on mid-to-long-term oncological safety cannot be made.

The primary limitations of this systematic review stem from the retrospective nature of the included studies. The small sample sizes and limited number of published papers may impact the precision and reliability of the pooled estimates. Additionally, a potential publication bias due to missing information in existing literature cannot be excluded. A publication bias analysis was not performed due to the preliminary nature of the available studies. Based on the IDEAL framework [32,33], which was developed to standardize the reporting method for surgical studies, three out of four case–control studies [19–21] can be classified as stage 2a (development), while the experience by Abaza and the case series by Rudnick are classified as stage 1 [12,27]. The preliminary nature of the studies included justifies the low quality of the evidence. Consequently, our results should be interpreted with caution, considering the likelihood of selection bias favoring highly selected candidates for DV-SP RAA. Further research with extended follow-up durations is necessary to enhance the robustness of these findings.

To date, this systematic review and pooled analysis represent the first comprehensive assessment of surgical and early postoperative outcomes for RAA performed using DV-SP. In addition to the well-documented benefits of robot-assisted surgery, the DV-SP offers further advantages, including enhanced dexterity for surgeons due to its wide range of motion, improved intracorporeal instrument triangulation, higher rates of SDD, and better cosmetic outcomes for patients. Our findings highlight the feasibility and safety of this technique, though further investigation is needed to assess long-term outcomes. Future studies should further explore the learning curve associated with DV-SP RAA for both experienced and novice console surgeons. Larger, randomized studies are needed and may lead to a more comprehensive understanding of the platform's clinical applications in the field of adrenal surgery.

5. Conclusions

This systematic review provides the most comprehensive evaluation to date of DV-SP surgery in the context of RAA, offering critical insights into its early outcomes. Despite the preliminary nature of the existing evidence and the need for further investigation, our findings affirm the feasibility, safety, and reproducibility of DV-SP RAA. The pooled data suggest that experienced robotic surgeons can seamlessly transition to DV-SP without compromising key surgical and oncological outcomes. However, the initial technical challenges and its extensive use remain important considerations. Further research is essential to delineate the full potential of DV-SP, particularly in managing complex cases such as bilateral masses and larger adenomas (>6 cm).

Author Contributions: Conceptualization and study design, G.R., F.Z., G.B. (Giovanni Betto), G.N., F.D.M.; data analysis and interpretation, G.R.; data collection, A.T., G.R., C.P., G.G., G.B. (Giorgia Baù), A.C., A.G., L.S., V.F., K.M., S.V., E.T.; writing—original draft preparation, G.R., F.Z.; review and editing, F.D.M., G.N., G.B. (Giovanni Betto), A.T., C.P., G.G., G.B. (Giorgia Baù), A.C., A.G., L.S., V.F., K.M., S.V., E.T.; supervision, F.Z. All authors have read and agreed to the published version of the manuscript.

Funding: This research received no external funding.

Institutional Review Board Statement: Ethical review and approval were not applicable for this literature review.

Informed Consent Statement: Not applicable.

Data Availability Statement: No new data has been created; all the data is available in the original manuscript included in the systematic review.

Conflicts of Interest: The authors declare no conflicts of interest.

References

1. Rowe, N.E.; Kumar, R.; Schieda, N.; Siddiqi, F.; McGregor, T.; McAlpine, K.; Violette, P.; Bathini, V.; Eng, M.; Izard, J. Diagnosis, Management, and Follow-Up of the Incidentally Discovered Adrenal Mass: CUA Guideline Endorsed by the AUA. *J. Urol.* **2023**, *210*, 590–599. [CrossRef] [PubMed]
2. Kahramangil, B.; Kose, E.; Remer, E.M.; Reynolds, J.P.; Stein, R.; Rini, B.; Siperstein, A.; Berber, E. A Modern Assessment of Cancer Risk in Adrenal Incidentalomas. *Ann. Surg.* **2022**, *275*, e238–e244. [CrossRef] [PubMed]
3. Corwin, M.T.; Navarro, S.M.; Malik, D.G.; Loehfelm, T.W.; Fananapazir, G.; Wilson, M.; Campbell, M.J. Differences in Growth Rate on CT of Adrenal Adenomas and Malignant Adrenal Nodules. *Am. J. Roentgenol.* **2019**, *213*, 632–636. [CrossRef] [PubMed]
4. Mihai, R. Open adrenalectomy. *Gland. Surg.* **2019**, *8*, S28–S35. [CrossRef]
5. Lal, G.; Duh, Q.-Y. Laparoscopic adrenalectomy—Indications and technique. *Surg. Oncol.* **2003**, *12*, 105–123. [CrossRef]
6. Feng, Z.; Feng, M.P.; Feng, D.P.; Solórzano, C.C. Robotic-assisted adrenalectomy using da Vinci Xi vs. Si: Are there differences? *J. Robot. Surg.* **2020**, *14*, 349–355. [CrossRef]
7. Piccoli, M.; Pecchini, F.; Serra, F.; Nigro, C.; Colli, G.; Gozzo, D.; Zirilli, L.; Madeo, B.; Rochira, V.; Mullineris, B. Robotic Versus Laparoscopic Adrenalectomy: Pluriannual Experience in a High-Volume Center Evaluating Indications and Results. *J. Laparoendosc. Adv. Surg. Technol.* **2021**, *31*, 375–381. [CrossRef]
8. Materazzi, G.; Rossi, L. Robot-assisted adrenalectomy: State of the art. *Updates Surg.* **2021**, *73*, 1131–1146. [CrossRef]
9. Nomine-Criqui, C.; Germain, A.; Ayav, A.; Bresler, L.; Brunaud, L. Robot-assisted adrenalectomy: Indications and drawbacks. *Updates Surg.* **2017**, *69*, 127–133. [CrossRef]
10. Morelli, L.; Tartaglia, D.; Bronzoni, J.; Palmeri, M.; Guadagni, S.; Di Franco, G.; Gennai, A.; Bianchini, M.; Bastiani, L.; Moglia, A.; et al. Robotic assisted versus pure laparoscopic surgery of the adrenal glands: A case-control study comparing surgical techniques. *Langenbecks Arch. Surg.* **2016**, *401*, 999–1006. [CrossRef]
11. Reitano, G.; Tumminello, A.; Ghaffar, U.; Saggionetto, G.; Taverna, A.; Mangiacavallo, F.; Ahmed, M.E.; Basourakos, S.P.; Carletti, F.; Minardi, D.; et al. Perioperative, Oncological, and Functional Outcomes of New Multiport Robotic Platforms in Urology: A Systematic Review and Meta-analysis. *Eur. Urol. Open Sci.* **2025**, *74*, 44–70. [CrossRef] [PubMed]
12. Abaza, R.; Murphy, C.; Bsatee, A.; Brown, D.H.; Martinez, O. Single-port Robotic Surgery Allows Same-day Discharge in Majority of Cases. *Urology* **2021**, *148*, 159–165. [CrossRef] [PubMed]
13. Beksac, A.T.; Zeinab, M.A.; Ferguson, E.; Kaviani, A.; Kaouk, J. Single-Port Extraperitoneal Robot Assisted Radical Prostatectomy—Description of Technique. *Urol. Video J.* **2022**, *15*, 100162. [CrossRef]
14. Abou Zeinab, M.; Kaviani, A.; Beksac, A.T.; Ferguson, E.; Kaouk, J. Single port transvesical simple prostatectomy: A minimally invasive technique in BPH management. *Urol. Video J.* **2022**, *14*, 100158. [CrossRef]

15. Francavilla, S.; Abern, M.R.; Dobbs, R.W.; Vigneswaran, H.T.; Talamini, S.; Antonelli, A.; Simeone, C.; Crivellaro, S. Single-Pc robot assisted partial nephrectomy: Initial experience and technique with the da Vinci Single-Port platform (IDEAL Phase *Minerva Urol. Nephrol.* **2022**, *74*, 216–224. [CrossRef]
16. Ganesan, V.; Goueli, R.; Rodriguez, D.; Hess, D.; Carmel, M. Single-port robotic-assisted laparoscopic sacrocolpopexy wi magnetic retraction: First experience using the SP da Vinci platform. *J. Robot. Surg.* **2020**, *14*, 753–758. [CrossRef]
17. Beksac, A.T.; Abou Zeinab, M.; Ferguson, E.; Kaviani, A.; Kaouk, J. Single-port retroperitoneal robotic pyeloplasty: Description technique. *Urol. Video J.* **2022**, *15*, 100178. [CrossRef]
18. Page, M.J.; McKenzie, J.E.; Bossuyt, P.M.; Boutron, I.; Hoffmann, T.C.; Mulrow, C.D.; Shamseer, L.; Tetzlaff, J.M.; Akl, E.A Brennan, S.E.; et al. The PRISMA 2020 statement: An updated guideline for reporting systematic reviews. *BMJ* **2021**, *372*, n7 [CrossRef]
19. Munn, Z.; Moola, S.; Lisy, K.; Riitano, D.; Tufanaru, C. Methodological guidance for systematic reviews of observation epidemiological studies reporting prevalence and cumulative incidence data. *Int. J. Evid. Based Healthc.* **2015**, *13*, 147–15 [CrossRef]
20. Dindo, D.; Demartines, N.; Clavien, P.-A. Classification of Surgical Complications. *Ann. Surg.* **2004**, *240*, 205–213. [CrossRef]
21. Sterne, J.A.; Hernán, M.A.; Reeves, B.C.; Savović, J.; Berkman, N.D.; Viswanathan, M.; Henry, D.; Altman, D.G.; Ansari, M.T Boutron, I.; et al. ROBINS-I: A tool for assessing risk of bias in non-randomised studies of interventions. *BMJ* **2016**, *355*, i491 [CrossRef] [PubMed]
22. Knoll, T.; Omar, M.I.; Maclennan, S.; Hernández, V.; Canfield, S.; Yuan, Y.; Bruins, M.; Marconi, L.; Van Poppel, H.; N'dow, J et al. Key Steps in Conducting Systematic Reviews for Underpinning Clinical Practice Guidelines: Methodology of the Europea Association of Urology. *Eur. Urol.* **2018**, *73*, 290–300. [CrossRef] [PubMed]
23. Sarkar, J.; Rashid, M. Visualizing Mean, Median, Mean Deviation, and Standard Deviation of a Set of Numbers. *Am. Stat.* **2016** *70*, 304–312. [CrossRef]
24. Lee, I.A.; Kim, J.K.; Kim, K.; Kang, S.-W.; Lee, J.; Jeong, J.J.; Nam, K.-H.; Chung, W.Y. Robotic Adrenalectomy Using the da Vinc SP Robotic System: Technical Feasibility Comparison with Single-Port Access Using the da Vinci Multi-arm Robotic System. *Ann Surg. Oncol.* **2022**, *29*, 3085–3092. [CrossRef]
25. Fang, A.M.; Fazendin, J.M.; Rais-Bahrami, S.; Porterfield, J.R. Comparison of Perioperative Outcomes Between Single-Port and Multi-Port Robotic Adrenalectomy. *Am. Surg.* **2023**, *89*, 1668–1672. [CrossRef]
26. Kim, B.-C.; Kwon, D.; Pak, S.J.; Cho, J.W.; Kim, W.W.; Sung, T.-Y.; Chung, K.-W.; Lee, Y.-M. Safety and feasibility of single-port surgery for posterior retroperitoneal adrenalectomy using the da Vinci SP robotic system: A retrospective cohort study. *Surg Endosc.* **2023**, *37*, 8269–8276. [CrossRef]
27. Rudnick, B.; Billah, M.S.; Nguyen, J.; Sheckley, F.; Ahmed, M. Surgical Technique and Perioperative Outcomes Following Single-Port Robotic Adrenalectomy: A Single Institutional Experience. *J. Endourol.* **2024**, *38*, 353–357. [CrossRef]
28. Esposito, G.; Mullineris, B.; Colli, G.; Curia, S.; Piccoli, M. Robotic Versus Laparoscopic Adrenalectomy for Adrenal Tumors: An Up-to-Date Meta-Analysis on Perioperative Outcomes. *Cancers* **2025**, *17*, 150. [CrossRef]
29. Moughnyeh, M.; Lindeman, B.; Porterfield, J.R.; Dream, S. Outpatient robot-assisted adrenalectomy: Is it safe? *Am. J. Surg.* **2020**, *220*, 296–297. [CrossRef]
30. Ortiz, D.I.; Findling, J.W.; Carroll, T.B.; Javorsky, B.R.; Carr, A.A.; Evans, D.B.; Yen, T.W.; Wang, T.S. Cosyntropin stimulation testing on postoperative day 1 allows for selective glucocorticoid replacement therapy after adrenalectomy for hypercortisolism: Results of a novel, multidisciplinary institutional protocol. *Surgery* **2016**, *159*, 259–266. [CrossRef]
31. Yilmaz, T.; Foster, R.; Hao, Y. Detecting Vital Signs with Wearable Wireless Sensors. *Sensors* **2010**, *10*, 10837–10862. [CrossRef] [PubMed]
32. McCulloch, P.; Altman, D.G.; Campbell, W.B.; Flum, D.R.; Glasziou, P.; Marshall, J.C.; Nicholl, J. No surgical innovation without evaluation: The IDEAL recommendations. *Lancet* **2009**, *374*, 1105–1112. [CrossRef] [PubMed]
33. Marcus, H.J.; Ramirez, P.T.; Khan, D.Z.; Layard Horsfall, H.; Hanrahan, J.G.; Williams, S.C.; Beard, D.J.; Bhat, R.; Catchpole, K.; Cook, A.; et al. The IDEAL framework for surgical robotics: Development, comparative evaluation and long-term monitoring. *Nat. Med.* **2024**, *30*, 61–75. [CrossRef] [PubMed]

MDPI AG
Grosspeteranlage 5
4052 Basel
Switzerland
Tel.: +41 61 683 77 34

Cancers Editorial Office
E-mail: cancers@mdpi.com
www.mdpi.com/journal/cancers

www.ingramcontent.com/pod-product-compliance
Lightning Source LLC
Chambersburg PA
CBHW062055220926
51850CB00010B/2775
9783725868667